TESTI

"You will enjoy this candid and insightful book, warts and all. As a fellow surgeon, '*Cutting It*' had me in stitches several times. It will inform and entertain both the public and those in the profession." – Lord Ribeiro.

"As elegantly written as it is witty and humane, Kevin Lafferty's '*Cutting It*' is a triumph. Not a word is wasted, not a page fails to entertain and enlighten. Lafferty's memoir of a life spent wielding a knife, in the best of ways, is easily one of the great books on surgery, that most paradoxical of human endeavours." – Alex Wade, writer and libel lawyer.

"Surgeons rescued me from the Grim Reaper more than once when I was a child. I've often wondered how they coped under such intense pressure, or how they would have reacted if I'd died on the operating table. Well, finally, I now have a good idea. Some scenes make you feel like you're wielding the scalpel yourself. Others will haunt you or tug at your heartstrings long after you've put the book down. '*Cutting It*' is on my Top 10 most-memorable books list: I guarantee you'll recommend it to your friends."
– Stephanie J. Hale BEM, author, broadcaster and journalist.

CUTTING IT

CUTTING IT

REAL-LIFE TALES OF GENERAL AND VASCULAR SURGERY

KEVIN LAFFERTY

POWERHOUSE
PUBLICATIONS

Powerhouse Publications
Suite 124. 94 London Road
Headington, Oxford
OX3 9FN

FOREWORD

As a colleague and friend for over 40 years, I am delighted to be writing the Foreword for this 'no-holds-barred' book on a surgical life, well-lived. Kevin Lafferty's reflections of events throughout his career are as crisp and clear as if they happened yesterday. The narrative is easy to read and dissects and explains the medical terms used through their Latin and Greek roots, for all to understand.

The loss of the generalist, can-do-all surgeon is a recurring theme. I recall working as a house surgeon for a urologist of international repute (Richard Turner Warwick), who because of his extensive training, could turn his expert hands to anything. Presented with a patient who had developed complications following a stomach operation done elsewhere, he proceeded to perform extensive corrective surgery that saved the patient's life. When asked how he – a specialist urologist – had done it, he replied, "One can always do the surgery, it's knowing why and when you should that matters." That same sentiment shines out through this book. Surgery is indeed a craft, but as the author shows, it requires practice, practice, practice, lots of experience, and a sixth sense to know when things are not right.

The author was an experienced and accomplished registrar when I took up my post as a consultant general surgeon in 1979, and he returned in 1987 to the same hospital group as a fellow consultant. Although appointed as a general and vascular surgeon, he and his vascular colleague took the specialty to new levels. But unlike many specialists he remained true to his general surgical roots, supporting trainees faced with emergency general surgical cases which threatened to overwhelm them, in the same way that he was helped during his own training.

There are few people in their lifetime who have a building named after them. Kevin Lafferty holds that distinction, and a postgraduate lecture theatre bears his name as testament to his persuasive fund-raising skills, educational ethos, and the esteem with which he is held. Even fewer pen a surgical masterpiece that is informative, witty and a must-read. This is not the only book by the author. '*A New Short Textbook of Surgery*' with Leonard Cotton and '*Concise Surgery*' with John Rennie, are both works that should grace every would-be surgeon's bookshelf.

You will enjoy this candid and insightful book, warts and all. As a fellow surgeon, '*Cutting It*' had me in stitches several times. It will inform and entertain both the public and those in the profession. It joins a list of recent publications by other surgeons: Atul Gawande, Henry Marsh and David Nott. Kevin Lafferty deserves to be added to that club of writers.

For those seeking to understand the craft of surgery and what makes surgeons tick – look no further.

Lord Ribeiro

CONTENTS

INTRODUCTION

When crafting a book of this nature, the moral, ethical and legal obligations of all doctors to protect the absolute privacy of patients is paramount. This constraint has proved to be troublesome when recounting true stories of individual people. Initially, I imagined an anecdote used as a single example of operations performed countrywide on hundreds or thousands of similar patients each year would provide sufficient privacy and anonymity. But then, I realised I would have to put my name to the piece, which narrows the odds of identification considerably. A pseudonym was rejected because it would negate the great affection, pride, and sometimes a little sadness, I continue feel for those patients mentioned. It might also imply I have something to hide, which I don't.

Consequently, where used, all patient names are fabricated, and to provide further protection, so are those of clinicians and other characters where necessary. Likewise, some of the lengthier disease-specific anecdotes are amalgams of two or more people with different social histories and physical attributes, rather than an individual patient who might – just might – be identifiable by themselves or others: I reasoned that a constructed persona would provide the mandatory privacy, but still allow the same degree of emotional involvement for the reader. An alternative approach would be to seek the written permission of every living patient to use their story, an impossible task given the lengthy timescales involved – even if I could recall their real names, which I genuinely can't. In any case, I have no wish or willingness to betray any patient's right to privacy, nor would it serve any purpose to do so.

Therefore, any foggy obfuscation you perceive in the narrative is either deliberate, or simply piss-poor writing – but neither diminishes the authenticity of the clinical tales.

In essence, this book is a timeline of my journey from schoolboy to consultant surgeon and beyond, using patients as instructive diversions. Along the way, you'll learn a useful amount of surgery, anatomy, physiology and pathology – but don't fret: it's easy reading and nowhere near degree-level. The aim is to inform, educate, and hopefully entertain those who are interested in the subject, and do it in a light-hearted easily understandable way.

That said, it's also turned out to be something of a love letter to surgery, and to the compulsive addiction of using your own hands to fix sick people. Although it's my letter, the content is not unique. Any surgeon with a long career in the craft could deliver a similar tribute and tell comparable bitter-sweet, hair-raising tales of derring-do. So, it's also a respectful nod to surgeons everywhere, and to our teachers, colleagues and co-workers. We've all ridden the same stomach-churning roller-coaster and know surgery is far more than a demanding job. Rather, it's a wonderfully captivating and, oftentimes, turbulent love affair. So, welcome to the ride. It's not always going to be heart-warming and uplifting, but that's life!

Before starting, it would be useful to describe a few of the stereotypes who pervade the medical profession and appear here and there in the text. As ever, they're a bit broad-brush and amusing, with a scintilla of truth, but free of any malice or disrespect. I make no apologies, for it is how it is.

Physicians – the pill-pushers – regard themselves as being intellectually superior demigods, and think all surgeons are thick, blood-lusting, psychopathic egomaniacs.

Surgeons – like me – think all physicians are anally retentive obsessive-compulsives who can't make a decision; and know, truly know, that cardiac surgeons really are psychopathic egomaniacs.

Orthopods – orthopaedic surgeons – think very little. They are muscle-bound rugby-playing primates with size-ten hands whose only interest is in bones, preferably broken ones.

Gasmen – anaesthetists – have nerves of steel, iced water for blood, and no idea how any of their general anaesthetic drugs work. Nor does anybody else, but at least a gasman knows an overdose of them will send you to sleep forever. They are the surgeon's friend when they're slick and quick, and a bane when they're slow. Surgeons and anaesthetists make great drinking partners.

General practitioners – GPs, family doctors – are good guys who do an impossibly difficult job and are unfairly rebuked for missing extremely rare conditions. Consultants never criticise GPs because it would be unprofessional: GPs are the main source of private patients.

Trick-cyclists – psychiatrists – are all mad. This is a widely held view, even among psychiatrists themselves, which somehow proves the point.

You might also appreciate some background information on me.

I'm the grandson of a Liverpool docker. My dad was one of seven siblings raised in the poverty and unemployment of that great maritime city during the depression of the 1920s and 30s. Like most working-class boys of his generation, he left school at fourteen with the same poor job prospects as his father: unskilled manual labour in the docks or on a merchant steamship plying the trade routes. For a few years, he worked in the docks as a fitter's mate and, had the status quo maintained, it's probable that a similar legacy awaited me. But the unlikely silver lining of Hitler's dark cloud intervened, providing a vastly different future for him and many others. Dad went to sea with the Royal Navy and not only survived but, somewhere along the way, became an apprentice marine engineer. Post-war, he swapped to the Merchant Navy, passed all the appropriate exams and finally returned to dry land as a chief engineer with transferable skills in industry. Mum was a factory girl with similar roots.

She spent the war loading munitions and dodging bombs, then afterwards loaded cigarettes at Ogden's tobacco factory while dodging amorous men. At least, that was her story, and from the twinkle in her eye, she enjoyed every liberating minute of it. I arrived in 1952, a baby boomer and the first of five kids.

Home was a small three-bedroom semi-detached on the outskirts of Liverpool, the first house either of my parents' families had ever owned. Back then, it was flanked by open countryside with trees, hedgerows, natural ponds and farmland, allowing me and the neighbouring young boomers unfettered access to a wild adventure playground. As a result, I developed a fascination with nature and science that remains with me to this day.

Catholic primary school furnished me with the eleven-plus, deep existential guilt, and a lifelong distrust in the credibility of nuns and priests. Palmer's grammar school for boys nurtured my scientific bent and erased any further interest in religion. Sixth form, and an outstanding teacher called Mr Twydell, gave me decent science A levels and pushed me into medicine. Sorry to disappoint, but there was no epiphany to save mankind, no family crisis, no tragic death or illness to set my heart on a career, and no other doctors in the family. I just fancied it, though there may have been subliminal coercion in the form of *Emergency – Ward 10* and *Dr Kildare*, my mother's favourite TV soaps.

Finally, I'm a lifelong supporter of Liverpool football club. It was inevitable. Dad regularly went to Anfield to stand on the Kop terraces for home games and, at the age of five or six, I'd be there with him, sitting on his shoulders and protected from harm by the surrounding fans. Hundreds, if not thousands of other boys were similarly inducted into the same creed. Innocent times.

And now, seemingly overnight, I've turned into a gnarled old man with a story to tell. So, hand me the knife and let's begin.

1

FIRST DEATH AND FIRST TEARS

Simon and Garfunkel's *Bridge over Troubled Water* topped the album charts for months on end; Mungo Jerry had a hit single with *In the Summertime*; the Apollo 13 crew told Houston they had a problem; the voting age fell from twenty-one to eighteen; Ted Heath's Conservative Party won the general election; the Beatles broke up; and the Woodstock festival, just a year before, had been the death knell of flower-powered hippie culture. The world now seemed to pause for a deep breath before jumping headlong into the confused, riotous, glam-rock, hard-rock, heavy-metal, skinhead and punk crazes of the new decade.

Girls wore embroidered Afghan coats, hot pants, mini, midi or maxi skirts with platform boots. Boys wore flared jeans and DIY tie-dyed grandfather vests or flowery shirts with absurdly large collars and a matching kipper tie. Suede desert boots, or leather ankle boots with a side-zip, adorned our feet; trainers were white plimsolls for use at the gym or tennis court. Clothes were tightly fitted and highly coloured; all hair was still long; everyone had a Carpenters LP in their collection but hid it because it was uncool, man; Jimi

Hendrix and Janis Joplin both died from a drug overdose and briefly became the coolest stiffs on the planet; every man in Britain watched *Top of the Pops* to drool over Pan's People; and Carnaby Street in London, the pulsating epicentre of all this trendy mania, was a ten-minute walk from The Middlesex Hospital, its medical school and nurses' home. Phew.

The year was 1970, and marked my transition from naïve pimply schoolboy to bewildered spotty undergraduate. I had the time of my life.

All the fun ended abruptly at the end of May 1975. I'd just turned twenty-three. The last clinicals of the final exams finished the previous afternoon and the results were due to be posted on the school noticeboard at two o'clock. What better way to spend the agonising wait than in the *King & Queen* across the street? It was an old-fashioned Victorian boozer with comfortable leather chairs, mahogany tables, oak-panelled walls, a good atmosphere, decent beer, and had been the watering hole and meeting place of medical students for at least a century.

The mood that lunchtime was uniquely sombre, neither a wake nor a wedding, but a demob party. Most of "our" year was there, sitting together in different groups wrought from flat-sharing, common sports, or amorous liaisons both temporary and permanent. We had spent almost a quarter of our young lives together, surrogate siblings sharing in all the adventure, excitement, heartache and fear that immature youth brings, each a member of the same extended family and changed forever by the experience. Whatever the day held for us academically, by the following morning our common kinship and close camaraderie would be gone, so the goodbyes, the handshakes and hugs were sincere and deeply felt. Many would leave immediately after the results were known, bags already packed, ready to be whisked away by elated or despondent parents, or would take a train home to face the same. The rest would be gone tomorrow, or hang around for a few days yet, waiting until the weekend. Our student days were over. Within a couple of months we'd all be working for a living, posted to hospitals all over Britain as pre-registration housemen for a year, the lowest of the low, and a compulsory requirement before the General Medical Council would add our names to the medical register as qualified doctors.

I sat at a table with my flatmates, four good men and true, all sipping beer with far less enthusiasm than I'd ever witnessed previously, a side effect of last night's celebrations. We were known as the King's Cross Crew after the locale of our damp vermin-infested digs, the top two floors of a three-storey terraced house at the back end of the main line station. Next to us were the Raveley Street Ratbags, a similarly hung-over bunch of guys from a less decrepit house near Tufnell Park, and arch-rivals in the home brewing, drunken bawdiness and partying stakes. We were all close mates and shared an exclusive undergraduate extra-curricular activity that brought us even closer. Later in life we realised it was probably the most important part of our training.

Not for us the supermarket shelf-stacking, postman, bartender, restaurant waiting, street cleaning and librarian jobs that others found to supplement their student grant. Or the lucrative visits to a nearby sperm bank: the genes of tall blond medical students were much in demand, despite grim warnings from the rest of us regarding blindness and the prospect of seeding the planet with countless numbers of genetically preordained habitual wankers.

For a year or more, the Crew and the Ratbags supplied unskilled labour to a small maintenance firm contracted to a large factory in suburban east London. Seven days a week, two of us would travel east and work for twelve hours, seven till seven, for a weekly wage of around £5 each in cash. That doesn't sound much now, but it equated to twice my weekly share of the rent and could buy a lot of beer, curry, and the occasional textbook. The roster depended on which clinical module each of us was doing at the time and who was most broke. In the core subjects of medicine and surgery our faces would be missed, but psychiatry, dermatology, ophthalmology, otorhinolaryngology (that's ear, nose and throat) and a whole load of other 'ologies were fair game. It was a continuous juggling act, but the financial and educational benefits far outweighed the risks of skiving off.

The man we worked for was Benny, a skinhead thug who was rumoured to have narrowly missed doing time for manslaughter. Not overly tall but built like a gorilla, he always wore white overalls next to his skin and had the voice and manner of a sergeant major. 'Fuckin' useless student cunts,' was his frequent appraisal. His corporal was Alf, a scrawny, greasy weasel of a man, always in the same filthy shirt and jeans, with long unkempt hair, a roll-up fag permanently stuck to his lower lip, and a mind like a sewer, 'I'm a bit of a ladies' man. If I can getta bit, I'll 'ave it.'

Benny and Alf were about ten years older than us, and lifelong buddies from the East End. We assumed they were small-time crooks, though no one was ever lunatic enough to ask. With Alf, as the devious brains of the two, and Benny, the front-man grunt, they could have stepped off the pages of a Dickens' novel, yet at heart, both were kindly rogues. Their firm had a grandiose name suggesting an international business, but as far as we knew consisted solely of Benny and Alf, and at any one time a brace of medical students. All the grotty, dirty, stinking, heavy maintenance jobs were ours to do: digging up pathways, laying them down, cleaning gutters, unblocking drains ... whatever. The work was unimportant: it was manual and mindless. What drew us back each day was the fascinating and entertaining company.

Wide-eyed twenty-one-year-old innocents being schooled in the real world of hard graft and hard knocks, where hard men toiled seven days a week to survive, bought *The Sun* for page three and the racing tips, and appearing before the beak, being on probation, or serving time inside was all part of normal life. As was a complete lack of financial security or planning, drunken brawls for fun on Saturday nights, petty theft, catching the clap, and casual infidelity. Alf was very approachable, regularly entertaining us with hilarious tales of illicit affairs, narrow escapes and numerous conquests, one of which had an unusual talent. She would hum a tune while giving him a blow job.

'What tune?' we asked, eager to learn.

'Well, anyfing really. She'd do requests, but me favourite was, *She'll be comin' roun' the mountain when she comes*. It's got a good beat to it when yer fink about it, ain't it?'

Due to his bulk and dark moods, we were wary of Benny, who always seemed to be a heartbeat-away from violence. Turning up late for work or failing to grasp the details of a task would stretch his reasoning and vocabulary, 'Yer can't be thick fuckin' cunts 'cos yer fuckin' students. So, yer must be just fuckin' cunts.'

The most instructive experience was how easily we became invisible to the rest of society. Covered in muck and sweat, with a shovel, pickaxe or jackhammer in our hands, men in suits and smartly dressed office girls passing by would make a point of ignoring us, or worse, cast fleeting scornful glances. Their body language was explicit: we were scum, third-class citizens not worthy of attention. For us, as tourists passing through, the contempt they showed was a lesson on the superficial nature of class structure and snobbery, but for Benny and Alf, children of Blitz-ravaged London from dirt-poor origins with a minimal education, it was an unfair attack on their livelihood, their life, and their wretched fate. To demonstrate our solidarity, we would join in and give the snobs two-fingers and a raspberry whenever their backs were turned, and then fall about in fits of laughter. Who needed 'ologies when you could learn people instead?

At our two tables, the mood and circumstances reflected the rest of the pub. For myself, I would wait for the weekend before going home, pass or fail. The prospect of living full-time with my parents again was unthinkable. After five years away, I was an alien bohemian compared to their staid, narrow existence, and a couple of days would be more than enough loving boredom. By way of escape, the following Monday I was setting out to drive to Greece for the summer months with a soccer teammate.

When word arrived the results were out, there was no sudden exodus to cross the road back to the medical school. The pub, in any case, would shut at two-thirty – no all-day opening in those days – and the results could wait another half-hour. We carried on drinking and chatting, savouring those last moments together, recalling tales of triumph and disaster, of Benny and Alf, and remarking on how smart and presentable we'd become. All the men had undergone a complete makeover as finals loomed near. Fashionably long hair, ponytails, beards, moustaches, expansive sideburns – grown and cultured for years – disappeared overnight. Short back and sides, with a clean shave, were the ticket to success in the clinicals and oral exams, plus a borrowed or hired suit and some boot polish. The dozen or so women in the year simply pulled their hair back, cut their nails, dumped the varnish and make-up, donned sensible shoes and wore longer skirts.

After the pub closed, we wandered in dribs and drabs to the noticeboard. Like everyone else, I first found my own name on the list (P), and then spent several minutes searching out those with (F) appended. There weren't many, with no surprises. After all the hard study, fitful sleep and nerve-shredding tension of the previous weeks, I expected euphoria. Instead, I felt numb, empty and drained. The five-year marathon was finally over.

Two months later, early morning on a sunny August 1st, tanned, fit and fiercely apprehensive, I took the Tube to Park Royal in west London and my first houseman post; chest medicine for six months. Sitting in the almost-deserted carriage while watching the dreary suburbs drift by, the realisation hit me like a hammer. This was it, my first proper job. Never again would I take the day off when I fancied, lay in bed until midday, then slob around for the afternoon. I was on the treadmill of full-time work. It was scary. And became a whole lot scarier when at eight o'clock my bleep squawked. I found a phone and dialled 0, the universal hospital switchboard number.

'On-call bleep check, thank you for answering,' the woman said mechanically.

'Hang on, what did you say?'

She repeated the mantra.

'Are you sure it's me on call?' All I'd done so far was visit admin, sign on, collect a white coat and take ownership of the offending bleep. It must be a mistake. 'This is my first time here. I've only just walked into the hospital.'

'Oh, sorry Dear, I forgot. It's change-over day, isn't it?

Everyone's new and it's the usual madness. What number's printed on that bleep you have?' I found four digits and told her. 'Well, my love, on my list that's the on-call medical houseman for today, so it must be you. Bye.'

Five minutes later, I was examining a "You are here" map of the hospital when the damn thing chirruped again. Heart pounding, I ran back along the corridor to the same wall-mounted phone. A different switchboard woman gave me a three-digit number to call. I dialled it, *please, not Casualty, pleeeze*. A man answered, 'Hello, is that my houseman?'

'Quite honestly, I've no idea.'

'Well, I've just spoken to the other chap and, by deduction, we worked out it wasn't him, so it must be you. Where are you?'

'Lost in an endless corridor.'

He chuckled, 'Yeah, so was I. Find exit "R", walk outside into the daylight and take the path directly in front of you; it's surrounded by lawns and flowerbeds. Keep going until you come to the last building on the left. I'll meet you at the door.'

The old Central Middlesex Hospital was a sprawling, largely one-storey affair, with supposedly the second-longest corridor in Britain. Most wards, offices, departments and sundry other buildings sprouted at right angles to the main thoroughfare. Other wards stood alone, separated from each other and the main building by acres of grass, a sure sign of a previous TB (tuberculosis/consumption) sanatorium, dating back to when it could only be treated with fresh air, exercise, healthy food, and rarely, surgery. All of which explains why the last building on the left turned out to be the chest ward.

The guy who met me was my registrar. It was his first day too, but he had the good sense to phone the previous incumbent – it comes with NHS experience – to get a handle on the job and arrive an hour or so before me. He was a graduate of St Bartholomew's Hospital, a Bart's man, by repute a supercilious breed, but I thought him pleasant enough. The day before, he'd been a senior house officer (SHO) at that same venerable institution, so was about two to three years senior than me. In my eyes, that ranked him somewhere between a guardian angel and God.

By now, it was eight-thirty. 'Seems this is our ward and I've done a quick round with one of the nurses. Far as I can tell, they're all TB, cancer or emphysema, so you spend the morning getting to know them and this afternoon we'll do a round together. Right now, though, I'm apparently due in clinic. See you here after lunch. Okay?' With that, he turned and was gone, marching off down the path I'd just trodden, back to the main hospital.

The chest unit became my domain for the next six months. It was two wards: the old-fashioned Nightingale type, male and female, with a good number of single rooms primarily for patients with "open" TB – those coughing up live bugs – who needed isolation from others until the triple-therapy antibiotics kicked in. There were about thirty patients in the wards at any one time, with a few more scattered on the Intensive Care Unit (ICU) or Coronary Care Unit (CCU), both housed in the main building. The on-call rota was one in two. Translated into harsh reality, that means there were only two medical housemen in the whole hospital. The rota was Monday, Wednesday, Friday, Saturday, Sunday, Tuesday, Thursday; repeat for six months. Casualty was the main source of work, day and night, supplemented by admissions from out-patient clinics run by the boss. During daylight hours, the other wards and care units were kept under control by their own teams, but at night they frequently called the houseman. The heavy week amounted to 144 hours in the hospital, the light week a mere 72. A bedroom was provided, but it was rare to get much sleep.

In retrospect, such a regime seems brutal, but it was the norm. Indeed, just a few years before, a single houseman would spend the whole six months living-in and being permanently on call. Some swore they never breathed fresh air or saw daylight the whole time. Life was hectic and sleep deprived, but I learned a great deal of medicine. And witnessed my first death.

It was an old woman in the CCU, late evening on my first Saturday on call. The West Indian Staff Nurse bleeped me because, 'She ain't doin' well.' After the bright lights of the main corridor, stepping into the unit through the industrial black-rubber swing doors was like entering a dark cave, forcing me to pause while my eyes adjusted to the sudden change. A deserted nurses' desk sat in the centre of the ward, illuminated by a barely glowing table lamp, reminiscent of an old-master painting with the whole canvas black as pitch save for a single candle pushing back the night. The only other source of light came from the far corner, where the curtain drawn around one bed radiated a soft yellow glow, punctuated by hunched shadows flitting behind its folds. Feeling my way through the darkness, I crept the length of the ward towards it, careful not to bump into unseen obstructions and disturb the other patients. Behind the curtain the wall light was turned on, and though less than ideal, I could see more clearly. It was a grim sight.

Propped semi-upright on three pillows lay a frail, wrinkled old lady, a thin faded nightdress drawn carelessly low over sagging empty breasts, with pure terror in her eyes. Frothy saliva streamed from the corners of her blue lips and, like a stranded fish, her gummy toothless mouth opened and closed rhythmically as she fought to gasp each desperate breath. Clinging to her sweat-drenched neck and chest, as if to restrain and prevent any possibility of escape, were long soggy rat-tails of thinning grey hair. The staff nurse was attempting to fix an oxygen mask on the woman's face, but she repeatedly palmed it away, arms flailing, head tossing. Even with my vast inexperience, I recognised she was *in extremis* and needed urgent, effective treatment. But I was in no position to give it.

The nurse, my usual source of guidance when suffering acute brain failure twinned with chronic ignorance, came from an agency and could barely tell me the patient's name, 'I only been here since eight and I's on my own.' The ragged set of notes on the table at the end of the bed were a foot thick and doubtless held seventy-five years of medical history, most of which would be useless to me. I quickly glanced through the first few, freshly written pages. She'd been admitted two days prior with an MI, pulmonary oedema and left heart failure. Treatment with diuretics, morphine and oxygen improved her condition initially, but there was no further information, no treatment plan, no guidance on resuscitation. It would be years before such things became standard protocol.

Let me explain the old lady's problem.

We all know the heart is a pump that circulates blood around the body, courtesy of William Harvey, an English physician who worked it out in 1628. In a resting adult, that's around five litres a minute (the total blood volume), or seventy heartbeats a minute at about seventy mls for each beat (70 x 70 = 4,900). What's less appreciated is that our mammalian heart is, in fact, two pumps. The right side collects deoxygenated blue blood returning from the body and pushes it through the lungs to pick up oxygen and turn scarlet; the left side collects the oxygenated blood from the lungs and pushes it out into the body once more. That's probably as far as school biology lessons took you.

But what would happen if the right side didn't pump as effectively as the left? Let's say the right heart only pumped out sixty instead of seventy mls each beat. The left heart has no option but to pump out, blamelessly, what it receives from the right via the lungs (sixty mls) and carries on regardless. So, where would the (10mls x 70 beats a minute = 700mls) un-pumped blood go? Well, it wouldn't "go" anywhere. What it does is to pool or back-up in the lowermost regions of the body, notably the legs when we are standing or sitting. Fluid – mainly water – then leaches out of the blood through the tiny peripheral capillaries and collects in the skin, fat and muscle to cause swelling, until the blood volume is reduced by seven hundred mls. The circulation then returns to a balanced state (albeit 4.3 litres instead of 5) but the lower body remains congested and swollen with fluid. No doubt, you have come across elderly friends or relatives with swollen feet, ankles and lower legs – most likely they had right heart failure. It used to be called dropsy, a shortened version of hydropsy, but the modern term is congestive cardiac failure. The excess tissue fluid is called oedema, from the Greek, "to swell", though in the USA it's edema. Your body and your physician will compensate for the fluid congestion by stimulating the kidneys to pee it out, so at least initially, right heart failure is a relatively benign condition. Left heart failure, the old lady's problem, is completely the opposite. In this case, fluid is dumped into the lungs rather than the legs, so you end up drowning in your own juice – pulmonary oedema – and it's deadly. Try breathing in the best part of a litre of water and you'll appreciate the problem.

In practice, the right heart tends to fail gradually, taking weeks or months before you notice the tight shoes and socks, or in severe cases, your belly distended with fluid, a condition called ascites, which rather imaginatively is Greek for "wineskin", and probably the origin of the phrase, "Drinking a skinful". Also, pure right or left heart failure is rare. It's usually a mixture with one or the other predominant.

The most common cause of heart failure is ischaemia (Greek again: "stopping blood") of the heart muscle, the result of furred-up coronary arteries. Initially, the oxygen-deprived heart muscle complains by cramping up and giving you crushing chest pain on exercise (called angina; Greek for "strangle"), which is nature's way of telling you to slow down. If the oxygen deprivation is severe enough, a portion of the heart muscle (myocardium) will die, and you will have suffered a heart attack, a coronary, a myocardial infarction, or MI. For a change, the word "infarct" derives from the Latin "to stuff", describing the appearance of swollen dead muscle, though I like to think if you've had an MI, both you and your heart are "stuffed": that portion of dead heart muscle won't contract, so the heart can't pump as effectively.

Treatment of ischaemic heart failure is best accomplished by fixing the diseased and narrowed coronary arteries with stents or bypass surgery. Like any muscle, the myocardium works better with an adequate blood supply and can pump harder when it needs to, without giving you angina or an MI. However, no amount of blood will resurrect dead muscle, so if damage has already occurred, it's probably for life. Broadly speaking, medical treatment of heart failure is pharmaceutical plumbing. Imagine your central heating system with a failing pump. Ideally, you simply replace the aged or crippled pump, but heart transplants are difficult to come by. So, make the pump more efficient by oiling it with drugs like Digoxin (derived from Foxglove; Digitalis) and similar modern preparations. Or, give it less work to do by shutting off some of the radiators, thereby reducing the volume of fluid it struggles with; diuretics (water tablets) are used nowadays but bloodletting was once common. Giving oxygen to breathe is akin to increasing the boiler thermostat; hotter water (more oxygen in the blood) means that old pump still delivers the same amount of heat (oxygen) even though it's shifting less fluid.

The Holy Grail would be to repair the damaged muscle with stem cells or implant a hi-tech pumping device with its own everlasting power source. It will happen, but such things weren't even on the horizon forty years ago.

The old girl in front of me had already received every tweak available. Her pump, her boiler, her entire system, was on its last legs. She was drowning in her own private swimming pool of pulmonary oedema and I had no idea how to help her. But I knew a man who did, and where to find him. 'I'll be back in five minutes with some help,' I whispered to the nurse.

My immediate superior that first-ever weekend on call was a smooth guy who insisted on being called Michael rather than Mike. In his fourth year at senior registrar level, he'd effectively finished training and was looking around for a consultant physician post. With at least ten years of on-call experience under his belt, he was bored rigid with the enforced tedium of hospital imprisonment. I found him where he'd been all evening, in the doctors' mess watching TV. As far as I knew, he rarely moved, but was happy to discuss a patient and gave advice readily enough, even though his long sighs were tinged with ennui. His special interest was endocrine medicine (that's hormones), so he could get enthusiastically animated over a diabetic coma or an Addisonian crisis (acute adrenal gland failure), though I'd yet to witness that side of his character.

The mess was a single large room with a two-bar electric fire, threadbare carpet, a couple of sofas and armchairs, and a long coffee table. A small kitchen area had a kettle, teabags, a huge tin of instant coffee, an open bag of sugar, half a loaf of stale white sliced bread and a small fridge containing rancid butter and sour milk. Littered with dirty cups, plates, old newspapers, medical journals and full ashtrays, it would be Monday morning before it saw a cleaner again. At close on midnight, Michael was alone, slumped in an armchair supporting one temple on his fist. The black and white TV, chained to the wall to curb its habit of escaping, was running an old movie, but his eyes were vacant and faraway. In retrospect, I recognise myself and every other senior registrar at that stage of our career. Worried about getting a consultant job, money, mortgage, wife and kids; sleep-deprived to a permanent zombie state but knowing any attempt at bed before two a.m. would be futile; and irritated by inexperienced juniors with seemingly no common sense. But there and then, I understood none of it.

All I knew was a sick old woman needed help, so I stood

in his line of sight and laid it on thick and straight, my arms and palms held out in supplication. 'There's a woman on CCU dying of left heart failure. I need your help. I need you to come and see her.'

His eyes lifted slowly to mine as he sighed, 'You're sure she's dying?'

Dumbly, I nodded a yes. And in that instant, hated him. Hated his cool suaveness, his emotionless response, his lack of urgency, his cufflinks and tightly knotted club tie, clean shirt, neat hair, shaved face, shiny shoes, his brilliant-white coat with nothing but a gold fountain pen in the breast pocket and an expensive stethoscope in the waist. In contrast, I felt grubby, unkempt, stubbly, ignorant, stupid, helpless, and weighed down by various handbooks, hammers, scopes and other tools expected of a simple houseman. And my coat was a dirty grey.

The truth is, he already knew the woman in question, primed by his peers to expect her demise. He would also have known every other critically ill patient in the whole medical unit. Mooching around the CCU, ITU and the wards, talking to the nurses, smelling out trouble and heading it off early is what every on-call senior registrar does first thing on Saturday and Sunday mornings, before breakfast, before Casualty gets going and drags them away, before a stupid houseman cocks something up. It was his job. In years to come, it would be my job. It had been every consultant's job. But he didn't let on, and I was a clueless rookie.

To my surprise he stood up. 'Let's go.'

Tall, with an easy elegance drawn from experience, he strolled unhurried and silent along the empty, endless corridor with me in tow. We halted at the CCU doors and he spoke again. 'Is it the woman in the far right-hand bed?'

'Yes,' I blabbered, eager to demonstrate any degree of efficiency. 'She's seventy-five, came in two days ag–'

He held up a hand to silence me. 'It's her fifth MI and she has no myocardium left. She's dying from end-stage cardiac failure. You could up the diuretics, but I'm afraid it'll do no good. It's probably kinder to up the morphine.'

I'd pushed him this far, but now it sounded as if he didn't want, or simply couldn't be bothered, to see her. 'Please come in and take a look. Tell me what to do.' I was frantic.

'I've just told you what to do.' He scanned my face for several long seconds, as if scrutinising it for signs of intelligent life. Then, his manner changed, and his voice softened. Perhaps it was pity, compassion, or more likely, simple surrender. Accustomed to giving orders to people a rung or two beneath him – people who were capable – he finally understood the poor sap standing in front of him was out of his depth. 'This is your first death, isn't it?'

'Yes. This is my first job. I only started – *When was it? It seemed like weeks* – last Thursday.'

He pushed open one of the rubber swing doors. 'After you.'

The nurse was where I'd left her behind the curtains. As we slid quietly into the cramped space, she lifted her gaze, slowly shook her head from side to side and whispered, 'She's goin', doctors.' All three of us stood at the foot of the bed, silent, reverent, watching the old lady. The oxygen mask was finally in position, but the flailing arms now lay limp at her side. Her previously heaving chest moved more slowly, the shallow efforts creating a gentle gurgling deep in her throat. Heavy-lidded restfulness replaced the terror in her eyes. Five minutes passed before she exhaled for the last time. And finally, mercifully, was still.

Michael took this as his cue for business as usual. 'Okay, now you need to examine her to make sure she's dead. Carotid pulse, respirations zero, palpate her chest for a heartbeat, pupil reflexes – you know the drill.'

I knew the drill alright, but I'd never done it before. I shuffled to the right side of the bed, Michael shifted to the left, the better to watch me. Pulling a pen torch from my breast pocket, I gently lifted her right eyelid with my left thumb … and was briefly stunned.

I'd examined lots of eyes – fully conscious, those in a drugged sleep, unconscious head injuries, insensate anaesthetised patients. They all have an intangible reflective quality that never previously registered with me. Yet in that moment, at some primal intuitive level, I recognised that sparkling characteristic was absent in this lady. The sensation made my skin crawl. It was like knocking at a front door but instinctively knowing no one's at home. Her eye, much like the house you're knocking at, looked normal but seemed empty and abandoned. A poet or religious person might say the light of life, or whatever you want to call it, had gone. I suspect a dead eye with a fixed dilated pupil doesn't reflect as much light as a living one, so it appears spookily unnatural. Whatever the reason, I've seen the same hundreds of times since: in patients, close friends and relatives, pet dogs, cats and horses. It always unsettles me.

Quickly moving on, hoping my pause was interpreted as careful examination, I flashed the torchlight at her pupil. No reaction, same on the left. No carotid pulse over one minute, no respiratory movement, no heartbeat to feel. Her still-warm chest was slicked with clammy sweat beneath my hand. I looked at Michael, 'She's dead.'

He nodded agreement and checked his expensive gold watch, 'Time of death, nineteen minutes after midnight.' The nurse made a note in ballpoint pen beneath the hem of her white apron, then excused herself to begin the paperwork. 'Do you happen to have an ophthalmoscope in one of those bulging pockets?' I did, and after a brief struggle, the white coat released it into my grip. 'Check out her retina,' he instructed.

Leaning over the woman's face, carefully focusing the scope on the back of her dead eye, felt like a gross invasion of some intimate privacy. 'Take a good look at the retinal artery and its branches. If you're lucky and in time, you'll see trucking. With no blood pressure, dissolved nitrogen comes out of solution and tiny elongated bubbles float about in the vessels. It's supposed to look like railroad trucks going along in a line and is a highly specific sign of death. You can only observe it in the retina of course, but it happens all over the body.'

Sure enough, the trucking sign was there. I never bothered to look for it again, though taught others to. For me, as I suspect for Michael, it would always be an intimacy too far.

Anisha was one of the patients I inherited from the previous houseman. At sixteen, she was slightly too old to be on a children's unit and considered too young to be accommodated on an adult ward, full of elderly coughing wheezing women, so sensible compromise provided her with one of the single rooms usually reserved for open TB cases. During her long internment, she transformed it into the equivalent of any teenage girl's bedroom, with a bedside rug, wall-posters, clothes, trinkets, and a transistor radio permanently tuned to pop music. I met her on my first ward round.

Waist-length raven hair with the sheen of gunmetal, huge chocolate-brown almond eyes, butterfly lashes, and a beguiling, brilliantly white smile, all wrapped in the slender, unaffected yet effortless grace young Asian girls seem blessed with, she enchanted everyone, including the boss and my registrar. Because she was such an unusually young patient, effectively still a child, the nurses called her "The Princess", and the name stuck. She had already endured weeks of heavy-duty intravenous antibiotics, but as the veins in her arms became inflamed and packed up one after another, she was swapped onto huge nausea-inducing tablets, coupled with painful thigh and buttock injections that made her eyes brim with tears. Yet her courage never faltered, her smile still lit the room, and her singsong voice always effused gratitude.

Every lunchtime and evening, her mother and other members of the family arrived with her meal, a variety of deliciously aromatic spicy food, held in stainless-steel tiffin boxes. Five years as a student had turned me into a hardened, cheap curry-house veteran, so such authentic homemade grub smelled, and soon tasted, like five-star cuisine. Unprompted, Anisha began saving a selection of delights in a spare tiffin and would present it to me after her visitors departed. No doubt, her mother also colluded in the plot designed to fatten me up.

Anisha, and many of the other patients, were part of the Ugandan-Asian exodus that arrived in England after the dictator Idi Amin drove them out in the early 1970s. Being so young and having attended the local schools, she spoke perfect English, whereas her elderly countrymen and women spoke Gujarati only. This presented me and the ward nurses with many problems. For example, how does a proud, eighty-year-old Indian gentleman explain to an Irish nurse that he hasn't had a shit for a week? Sister tried to get him to talk to Anisha, but he took one look and fled back to his bed; a girl young enough to be his great granddaughter would never hear of his embarrassing problem. Finally, after much hand waving, pointing, posturing and farting noises on both sides, I understood the old man's predicament and prescribed a laxative. But the incident gave me an idea. A list of English words was presented to Anisha: "cough", "blood", "pain", "pus", "phlegm", "allergy", "tuberculosis", "infection", "constipation" and many others. Could she give us phonetic Gujarati translations? 'Yes,' she frowned, 'But what is this p-h-l-e-g-m?' Our accents were bad yet passable, and armed with her list we could at least communicate at a basic level. "Are you coughing up red blood or yellow pus? Where is the pain?" Within a week, I'd memorised the phrases but kept a copy in my burgeoning white coat. Another was pinned to the nurses' noticeboard.

For many weeks of my first houseman post, Anisha was an ever-present part of my daily work. Other patients came and went, either home (those with TB, sarcoidosis, acute asthma) or to the mortuary (terminal lung cancer), but she was a constant feature – and what's more, she was getting better. Her blood cultures were clearing, erratic temperature stabilising, weight and appetite increasing, exercise tolerance improving. 'Another week or two of antibiotics,' the boss said, 'Then, she can go home.'

The dark slate sky was spitting horizontal rain when I arrived on the ward one dank early-winter morning. As usual, when I'd not been on call the previous night, I made straight for the nurses' station. It was a little after seven-thirty, the night crew were handing over to the day shift and they were all huddled around the desk. 'Anything for me?' A list of admin jobs needed doing and I learned which patients were to be chastised for being caught outside in the middle of the night having a crafty fag, but there was nothing else of significance. Then, I overheard someone report the Princess was having a lie-in that morning. It immediately struck me as odd. 'What do you mean?' I butted in. 'She's still asleep,' came the shoulder-shrugging reply, 'So we didn't disturb her.' A small "Ding!" sounded in my head. It's not unknown for patients to be found dead in bed on morning nurses' rounds. The discovery is usually followed by a Crash Call and the rapid arrival of a resus team who diagnose a cold body, stiff with rigor mortis.

Seconds later, I was at Anisha's bedside. She appeared to be sleeping peacefully on her right side, the blanket over her chest rising and falling with each gentle breath. Crouching down to stare at her face, I put a hand to her left shoulder, felt reassuring warmth through the fabric of her pyjamas, and gently shook her. Any moment now, those big brown eyes would open, at first startled, and then bemused. But they didn't. Wouldn't. 'Anisha, wake up,' I shook her again, hard, then harder still. Nothing. By now my heart was thumping in alarm and I was whispering to myself, *'Don't do this to me now, kid. C'mon, wake up, WAKE UP!'*

I pushed her body to a semi-flat position. Her head rolled with it like a rag doll, but she remained unconscious. *She's out of it. Jeez, what's going on here?* It wasn't panic I felt, but dread concern for this beautiful child. *Do your job and examine her properly.* Dragging the top sheet and blanket from the bed, I threw them into a corner, then pushed her hips and legs until she was fully flat. Her breathing remained calm and regular. For all the world, she was lying there in pyjamas, fast asleep, warm, pulse normal. The day before, she'd looked the same, but conscious, awake, alert, smiling, talkative. Alive. Instinct and training made me start at the top in order to work downwards in a methodical way. With my thumbs, I gently lifted both her eyelids. The right pupil was dilated, blown out, the left normal. *No, no, no.* Missing everything else, I dived to her feet. Dragging my thumbnail over the sole of her right foot made the big toe flex and point down towards the bottom end of the bed, a normal response. On the left it went up. *Oh shit, not to her. This can't be happening to her.*

Anisha was initially admitted with a PUO – Pyrexia of Unknown Origin – which is exactly what it states, a persistently higher temperature than is normal, the cause of which is unidentified. Because of her ethnic origin and the fact that common things, are indeed, common, she was originally labelled as having TB somewhere, even though her chest X-ray was clear. Tuberculosis, named because of the nodules – tubercles – of cheesy pus it produces, often presents with a PUO, night sweats, and chronic ill-health, which explained her accommodation on the chest ward. But it turned out she didn't have TB. Indeed, at her age and attending school in England, she'd probably had a BCG vaccination and been protected.

What she did have was streptococcus germs in her blood cultures and a heart murmur which, along with other minor physical signs, made the diagnosis of what was at that time called subacute bacterial endocarditis, or SBE. Put simply, a common sore throat bug had somehow entered her bloodstream, then set up home on the aortic valve inside her heart. The term "subacute" refers to the insidious, slow onset of symptoms as opposed to the acute variety caused by more virulent organisms. Before the advent of antibiotics, any form of bacterial endocarditis was invariably fatal.

Having billions of bacteria growing like mildew on a heart valve causes two main problems. First, the component flaps of tissue get eaten away, which produces a leaky valve with a telltale murmur and eventual heart failure. And second, the bloodstream is continually flushed with bacteria washing off the valve, resulting in fever and general debilitation from septic blood, or septicaemia. In addition, if a particularly large – though still microscopic – clump of bacteria detaches from the valve, it can lodge in a small artery or capillary anywhere in the body, causing an obstruction to the blood flow. Depending on where the clump ends up, it produces minor problems such as a tender muscle, a small skin blemish, and tiny splinter-like lesions seen beneath the fingernails. Or something more serious.

Anisha had clearly suffered a huge brain injury. At some stage, a bacterial clump must have lodged somewhere in the right side of her brain. Ordinarily, this might have caused a stroke, but if it was small enough, or in a region where it produced no symptoms, she wouldn't have noticed anything. But the bacteria continued to grow and multiply, slowly eroding the wall of the artery until it burst, filling her skull with high-pressure blood. The blown right pupil and the up-going left big toe told me so. To this day, I hope it all happened in her sleep. And that it was quick.

I bleeped my registrar, wishing to all that's Holy he was

already in the hospital. He answered within seconds. 'What's up?'

'The Princess has stroked out.'

'I'm on my way.'

Ten minutes later, he confirmed the diagnosis. A stunned expression and glistening eyes betrayed his own feelings, yet in me he recognised utter despair. 'Go get yourself a coffee and leave this to me. I'll tell the boss and have her transferred to the ITU.'

She was put on a ventilator and given large doses of steroids in a vain attempt to decrease the inevitable brain swelling. By the next day, both her pupils were fixed and dilated, and she'd stopped breathing for herself. The neurosurgeons agreed she was brain dead and the boss himself turned off the ventilator. Minutes later, her oxygen-starved heart stopped beating and the heart monitor flat-lined. After months of medically induced torment, The Princess, the sweet, adorable golden child, was dead.

I left the ITU, went to the chest ward, parked my bleep and white coat at the nurses' desk and told them I'd be back in an hour. Then, I walked out of the hospital, found a nearby public park, sat on a bench in the pouring rain, dropped my head into my hands, and let loose a raging tsunami cocktail of anger, guilt, shame, blame, sorrow, regret, and injustice, stirred with desolate grief, until my eyes ran dry. It was the first, and only time, I ever shed tears over the death of a patient.

I can't say exactly why that should be. Maybe it was because I was young, inexperienced, vulnerable to my own emotions, held an immature faith in the power of medicine to conquer all, and never before had encountered such unspeakable tragedy. Possibly in that moment I grew up, learnt all the hard lessons in one colossal hit, and developed a protective shell to forever shield me from future hurt. Or, perhaps, no other death would ever touch me so deeply.

Recounting this tale illustrates how primitive diagnostic medicine was in 1975. Ultrasound scanning was still experimental, echocardiograms unheard of, CT (Computerised Tomography) and MRI (Magnetic Resonance Imaging) belonged to a future digital world. We had stethoscopes and X-rays. Bacterial endocarditis would now be diagnosed with a two-minute painless bedside scan, modern antibiotics delivered via a long-term central venous catheter, and the diseased aortic valve replaced with a prosthesis. But back then, open-heart surgery in the UK was still in its infancy and I doubt such a radical intervention would have been considered. Anisha was born just ten years too early to survive.

2

THE LITTLE GIRL
WHO LOST HER SPLEEN

Monday morning, seven o'clock, towards the end of my six-month surgical houseman post. I'd had the weekend off, so the first job of the day was a quick check of the wards to look for any of my patients with the O sign: unconscious, with an open mouth. Or worse, the Q sign: same as the O sign, but with the tongue hanging out to one side and no pulse. They were all fine. Good – I'd do a proper round after the operating list. My second job was to see the pre-ops, mark the site and side of the operation with a "cut here" arrow in black felt-tip pen, then fill in the consent form and have them sign it. Then, I was free to go to theatre and get my hands dirty. If there was time, I might even be let loose on another hernia.

No doubt about it, I was hooked on surgery. Made for it. As a student, many of my classmates hated it, declaring it either tediously boring or nausea-inducing, machismo-driven butchery. For me it seemed dramatic, electrifying and alluringly clever, but my inferior rank made me an outsider on the touchline looking in. Now, working within the discipline and an integral part of a surgical team, I found people on my wavelength, prepared to make decisions and act on them rather than order a few more tests – just in case – then get another opinion – again, just in case – and generally faff about in the pseudo-intellectual, self-important manner of physicians, all the while conducting endless mind-numbing ward rounds which could last for days. Surgeons simply got on with it. No fuss, no macho characters, just equally intelligent people wanting to get the job done, immediately when necessary, and possessing the skills to do it. I'd found my niche and my kindred spirits. What's more, they recognised the same in me.

A few weeks earlier, I'd been allowed to do my first solo appendix on a teenage lad. Diagnosed, admitted, operated, then discharged him a few days later. Cured with my own hands. All my own work. Mind-blowing, magical, better than ... Whoa ... hold on, let's not get too carried away. And yet, given the choice between a roll in the sheets and another appendix to fix? I was contemplating the question when the bleep squealed. Casualty wanted me. Urgently.

She was a scrawny little kid, flat on her back with no pillow, arms spread wide, stripped naked but for teddy-bear print knickers. The adult-sized trolley made her look small and vulnerable. Her clothes were in a small, sad heap on the floor beneath it, a grubby white tee shirt, denim shorts made from cut-off jeans, and bubble-gum pink plastic sandals, all hastily thrown where they lay. I noted the clean, bob-cut dark hair, the dirty hands, scuffed knees, tanned limbs, and imagined a tomboy. At nine in the morning, the emergency resuscitation room was flooded with warm sunlight through the high-set windows, and somewhere further down the corridor a radio was playing *Don't Go Breaking My Heart*, again. It was the endless sweltering summer of 1976, with Elton John and Kiki Dee supplying the equally endless soundtrack. Kids everywhere, free of school and not housebound by rain, were getting into the usual scrapes with cuts, bruises, sprains, green-stick fractures, dislocated elbows and head injuries. But this one was different. No tears, no frantic screaming for Mummy, no kicking, no wriggling. No movement at all. And her belly was swollen. This one was collapsed and in big trouble.

The specific medical term for this is shock; a failing blood circulation. An example of a layman's perception of shock would be a wife discovering her husband of twenty-years in bed with the man from next door. She might well be shocked, and at the furthest extreme, homicidal, but she wouldn't be *in* shock. If, however, she fainted and fell to the floor, it would be classed as neurogenic or nervous shock, the circulatory failure evidenced by lack of blood to her brain rendering her unconscious, albeit temporarily. Overwhelming infection (septic shock), heart problems (cardiogenic shock) and allergic reactions (anaphylactic shock) also cause circulatory failure.

Shock is a bad thing. The brain demands a constant and plentiful supply of oxygen and glucose delivered at a decent pressure, so the lights go out very promptly if the heart misses just a few beats or blood pools in the legs, as in the betrayed wife. Poor circulation to the lungs means the blood and therefore every cell in the body gets deprived of oxygen, which in turn leads to a further fall in blood pressure, and deeper shock. Kidneys are almost as temperamental as the brain, quickly getting into a hissy fit without a good filtration pressure, but they reveal their displeasure in a less dramatic way. It may be many hours before you or your doctor realise you've stopped peeing and your kidneys are knackered. Unless treated and reversed, the downward spiral of a failing blood circulation will generally lead to all organs calling in sick. Or not calling at all. And that's a really bad thing.

The sort of shock a surgeon usually encounters is caused by bleeding (haemorrhagic shock). The physiology is gratifyingly simple; if there's nothing in the pipes to circulate, there's no circulation. An adult man of average size contains five litres of blood. By the time he bleeds out two litres, less than half the total, he'll be comatose and hearing the distant lullaby of his kidneys singing *Goodnight Vienna*. The little girl on the trolley would have a normal blood volume of around two litres or less, so she wouldn't have to spill much for it to be life-threatening. As we say in the trade, the kid was totally clapped out. Sometimes, we say dying.

Above the oxygen mask, her eyelids were half-shut – neither awake nor asleep, but unconscious; the eyes glassy and vacant, beyond pain, beyond fear, beyond caring. A sheen of sweat glistened on her body and she panted like an exhausted dog. The heart rate monitor showed a super-fast 150 in luminous green digits. A nurse tried to get a blood pressure reading from a cuff on the girl's skinny left arm, 'I make it seventy at best,' but her voice, overly loud due to the stethoscope blocking her ears, was shrill with panic. On the other side of the trolley, the Casualty consultant was just finishing a cut-down insertion of an intra-venous line into the long saphenous vein, at the point where it reliably and conveniently crosses the ankle joint. I knew this to be a desperate measure, it meant all the peripheral veins were shut down and empty through lack of blood. Now, he squeezed the transparent bag of saline attached to the line, pushed a few rapid fistfuls of fluid into the bloodstream and opened the drip to full on. It would do for now, but what she really needed was blood.

Turning to face me, he must have read my mind. 'Six units being cross-matched ...' he checked the wall clock, 'be about thirty minutes. I told the lab to pull their fingers out. In the meantime, some O-neg's on the way.' He flicked his head toward the kid, 'Now, you examine her belly while I tell you the story.' Tall, middle-aged and slightly camp, with a reputation for abruptness bordering on rude, he was also slick, quick and talented. He'd overseen Casualty for years. I'd been there for all of twenty seconds.

'Ten-year-old girl, no previous history of note ...' he began.

Bending down, I felt her abdomen. It was tightly swollen, but she didn't flinch to my touch.

'Fell off a pushbike about an hour ago ...'

There was a graze on her left flank I'd not noticed before. On deeper palpation, the right side was soft and yielding, the left felt rock-solid in comparison.

'Okay for ten to fifteen minutes. Didn't even cry, a right little toughie. Then, she fainted and couldn't stand up. Mum dialled 999 ...'

Running diagonally across her abdomen was a line of firmness, hard above, soft below. I could feel two notches along the edge of the firm line.

'The ambulance crew found her unresponsive and blue-lighted her here ...'

Christ Almighty, how come her spleen's so big? The notches were the giveaway. A final check, definitely spleen, but this time she squirmed with discomfort. The saline infusion was increasing the circulation to her brain, but it wouldn't last for long. Salted water doesn't carry enough oxygen.

'And you know the rest,' he finished.

I stood upright again, recognising the scenario as an impromptu teaching session, or a test. 'She's in shock and her spleen's the size of a rugby ball.'

'Jolly good,' he drawled the words. 'Where's your boss?'

'He's in theatre with the registrar doing a list. That's why I'm here instead of the reg'.'

'Even better. So, what are you going to do now?' He put on a false smile.

'Go up to theatres and talk to him. She's ruptured her spleen and needs surgery.'

'Excellent. But tell him this: because it's so urgent, I'll push the trolley into the lift and bring her up there myself. And tell him it's not ruptured yet. Right now, it's a sub-capsular haematoma.'

Before we go any further, I need to tell you some facts.

If you have a backbone, you have a spleen. All vertebrates do, including fish and amphibians, though theirs is harder to spot. In us, it's hidden away in the top left-hand corner of our belly, and as far back as it can get, so even in humans, it's not easy. Think of where your parents hid the birthday and Christmas presents in the bedroom wardrobe when you were a kid and you'll get the idea. But instead of spare blankets and pillows, our spleen is stuffed behind the colon and stomach with the left kidney beneath. Make a fist with your left hand. That's the size of your spleen. Now, place your fist on the back of the left side of your chest. You'll have to rotate your wrist and shoulder, but when you've reached as far as you comfortably can, your spleen will be as close to your fist as it's ever going to get. That's how far back it is, or if you're unfortunate enough to be flat on an operating table, how deep.

Fundamentally, the spleen is a filter. Like the oil filter on your car engine trapping harmful debris and metallic particles, the spleen sieves the blood of ageing red cells, bacteria and other crud. In addition, unlike an inert oil filter, it contributes to your general well-being by producing white cells primed for defence and has a role in re-cycling iron. In common with other offal – liver and kidney will come to mind – the spleen is a collection of highly specialist cells with miles of small delicate blood vessels, all held together by a transparent sheet of tissue called "the capsule". The tissue of the capsule is called peritoneum (Greek: *peritonos*, stretched round), and covers everything inside the abdomen. It's basically organic cling film and about as flimsy, though if I had to choose, cling film has the edge. If you've ever prepared a lamb's kidney for the frying pan, the recipe always includes instructions to remove the membrane around it – that's the capsule. Thin, isn't it? Now imagine that kidney in life, pink and pulsating with a good blood supply, enclosed in its capsule, and give it a whack with a stick. If the blow is blunt and gentle enough, the capsule will stay intact, but the kidney itself will shatter and bleed. The blood will pool within and be contained by the capsule – a sub-capsular bleed – and because blood which isn't moving tends to clot, the correct description is a sub-capsular haematoma. Now, you understand the Casualty consultant's diagnosis.

Because the spleen is so fragile, evolution has ensured it is well-protected from injury. The left lower ribs shield its rear, left side and frontal approaches, and it's so far away from the right side as not to matter. Indeed, so closely are the ribs applied, the surface of the spleen often has characteristic indentations made by them – so-called notches. In addition, and this is another evolutionary adaptation, although the substantial pencil-thick splenic artery spans a distance of three or four inches, it is remarkably wriggly and tortuous, so if pulled straight would double its length. In other words, the artery is effectively a spring or bungee cord, allowing the spleen to move sideways and up and down under the influence of high acceleration forces, such as falls, rugby tackles and car crashes, without being torn away from its blood supply.

Because of this defensive armoury, it's surprisingly

difficult to damage a normal spleen. An assailant sticking a long knife in the correct place could do it, but that's quite rare. A clumsy surgeon already working within the abdomen can accidentally do it, which, believe me, is not uncommon. But the most assured way is massive blunt trauma to the left side, such as from a bus or high fall, which invariably fractures the ribs and crushes the ribcage, pushing sharp fragments of bone through the lung, the diaphragm, and most pertinent, into the capsule of the spleen and the sponge of blood vessels within. However, and you may have already formed the same conclusion, after being run over by a bus or fallen from a good height, a ruptured spleen is probably the least of your problems. You're most likely already dead.

So, given the facts, a tiny kid falling off her pushbike simply didn't fit the bill for a damaged spleen.

I left Casualty and ran full pelt up the stairs to theatres. Being young and fit, it was quicker than waiting for the lift – a slow, industrial contraption with manual sliding scissor gates designed to amputate fingers and ensure nurses in uniform stood modestly at the back. A hurried change into theatre greens and I was trotting along the corridor to operating room five. After the heat, sweat and urgency outside, the air conditioning made my skin prickle and cooled my head. This needed to be good. For the girl's sake, I was about to demand a halt to the routine list: two hernias – surgeons like to start with a few easy operations as a sort of warm-up exercise – a duodenal ulcer, then a gall bladder, then ...

I pushed the swing-door open. Anaesthetist, scrub nurse, circulating nurses, medical students and registrar, all heads turned to me. The boss though, kept his eyes down and his hands working. He seemed to be finishing off the first hernia. Good.

'Er, Mr Hawes,' I tried to sound cool and professional. 'There's a ten-year-old girl in Casualty who urgently needs her spleen out.' I ran through the history and events downstairs, finishing with, 'She'll be up here any minute in the direct lift, and you're the only general surgeon in the department.'

That was true. There were orthopods, gynaecologists, urologists and the ENT boys, but none of them were a blind bit of use for my needs. Dick Hawes – a reasonable man of few words, a patient teacher, a calm surgeon not known for tantrums or venomous outbursts – turned his gaze away from his hands and the hernia wound to the anaesthetist at the head of the table, and slowly raised an eyebrow. She in turn paused for a second, then nodded approval.

Anna Kirkby was short, trim, and efficient, a quality that seems to come easily to professional women with a bunch of young children at home. In common with many trainee Australian doctors in the 1960s and 70s, she arrived in England to gain further experience in her chosen specialty. Being a junior anaesthetist, she came to "gas the poms" for a year or two, then almost inevitably, married a British doctor and stayed here, finishing her training in a succession of London teaching hospitals.

Kirkby and Hawes were a smooth double act. NHS or private, she anaesthetised all his patients and had done for years. They knew each other's strengths and weaknesses, likes and dislikes, unspoken thoughts. What's more, having done a stint at Great Ormond Street, she was a genius with children.

'Right,' speaking with a loud Ozzy twang to no one in particular, 'Get that next hernia out of the anaesthetic room and park him in recovery. When the kid gets here, stick her in there. If she's that crook, I'll need some time and space to do a few things.'

Anyone who has had an operation will fully understand, but for those who are not so unlucky, I'll translate. The anaesthetic room is the annexe to any main operating theatre. In there, the anaesthetist is surrounded by cabinets full of drugs, tubes, cannulas, bags and bottles of intravenous fluids, and other paraphernalia. There's also another anaesthetic machine with medical gases, a mechanical ventilator, and appropriate dials, whistles and flashing lights. To keep a routine operating schedule running on time, the next patient on a list should be in the anaesthetic room before the previous one comes off the operating table. That way, the anaesthetist can wake the patient "on the table" and go straight to the annexe to gas the next. Unfortunately for him, the next on that day was expecting a hernia repair. Instead, his trolley would be pushed to a corner of the large suite where patients recover from their anaesthetic, and there he would wait, indefinitely.

When the girl was wheeled from the anaesthetic room and gently lifted onto the operating table under the dazzlingly bright "flying saucer" light, her belly resembled a balloon at the point of bursting. By then, there was an intravenous line in her left arm with a bag of blood, at last, running through it, a urinary catheter in her bladder but nothing trickling into the polythene bag attached, and an endotracheal tube in her mouth supplying anaesthetic vapours and oxygen to her lungs. The drip into the ankle vein was also connected to a second blood bag. Blood, and yet more precious blood, pouring in.

Dick Hawes was already scrubbed, gloved and gowned, and had been for twenty minutes, silently prowling the length and breadth of the operating room in white rubber boots, arms crossed to keep his gloves sterile and away from his mask, chin on chest as if deep in thought. An outside observer might envisage such restless contemplation in a surgeon to be a way of mentally preparing for the forthcoming battle to save a life. A quiet prayer perhaps, to guide his hands towards a successful outcome, or an imaginary rehearsal of the complex anatomy to conquer. The observer, however, would be very wide of the mark.

Such praiseworthy soul-searching is a fantasy of Hollywood scriptwriters and TV soaps. An on-screen airline captain would never be routinely scripted to begin praying for guidance as he opened the throttles for take-off, yet medics, and particularly surgeons, often are. Self-doubt has no place in the psyche of either a consultant surgeon or an airline captain because it would be an acknowledgement of poor training, inexperience and inability to do the job. Dick Hawes' prowling was probably no more than irritation at having his routine list decimated, a row with his wife, his football team's recent poor form, or a thousand other things. But never doubt in his own ability. Of course, he may have been preparing himself to tell the parents their precious little girl was dead.

The scrub nurse, an experienced senior sister, stood in one corner similarly dressed, but her gloved hands rested, knuckles down, on the sterile green towel covering her instrument tray. She stared vacantly at the floor, remembering which instruments would be required, in what order, and hoping she hadn't forgotten any.

The registrar was also scrubbed and spoke quietly to me, 'I doubt we'll get through the rest of the list. Depending on how long this takes, you're going to have to cancel at least one patient and tell them I'll bump them on to next week.'

'Okay, will do. But I want to watch this first.'

'No problem.'

Dr Kirkby and her assistant, an anaesthetic registrar dragged from a tedious orthopaedic list next door to help, spent a few minutes adjusting tubes, dials and flowmeters. Then, they conferred, 'Happy?' It wasn't an idle question. Kirkby was ensuring nothing had been overlooked in the frantic hurry to deliver the child to the operating table in a fit enough state to have some chance of getting through the surgery. The registrar, another experienced woman, scanned their work with a keen eye, 'She's as good as she's going to get.'

Kirkby turned to Hawes who now stopped his pacing.

'Okay, Dick, you can have her, but make it quick. We're only just holding on here.'

Within a minute, the girl's swollen abdomen was the only thing exposed, the rest of her body covered in sterile green drapes. The skin, still wet from antiseptic prep solution, glistened pearly white in the glare of the overhead light. Hawes held out his hand, 'Knife.' The scrub nurse slapped the handle of the scalpel into his palm. Closing his fingers around it, he murmured to the registrar on the opposite side of the table, 'Get the sucker ready.' Without pause, he skated the blade down the centre of her belly from sternum to pubis (top to bottom), neatly skirting the umbilicus. The skin and thin coating of yellow fat parted easily. There was some bleeding, which ordinarily he would have cauterised (Greek: branding iron) with electro-diathermy (Latin: through heat) forceps, but the blood loss was paltry in comparison to what was happening deeper inside, so he ignored it. The next layer was the midline tendon holding the abdominal muscles together. He started at the top end because underneath would be liver and stomach, no bulging bowel which is so easily and inadvertently pierced. Still using the scalpel blade but now the pointed tip, he deftly parted the tough tendrils of tissue until a bubble of delicate peritoneum pouted toward the ceiling. It was plum-coloured instead of clear, a sure telltale of a belly full of blood. Handing the knife back to Sister, blade down handle first, he barked, 'Scissors.' Twenty seconds gone.

With the scissors in his right hand, but holding them

backwards with the blades pointing to his wrist, he placed the tip of the lower blade on the pulp of his left index finger and plunged both through the bubble of peritoneum. Dark watery blood fountained out. The registrar put the tip of the sucker at the well-head to do its work, but it was a hopeless task, blood poured over the drapes in rivers and dripped to the floor. Meanwhile, Hawes slit open the length of the incision by simply pushing the partly opened blades of the scissors along the midline tendon, all the while protecting the underlying coils of gut with his index finger at first, and finally his whole hand. It was like watching a decorator cut wallpaper. Another ten seconds.

Hawes passed the scissors back to the sister and immediately pushed his right hand as far as the wrist into the belly, displacing a further scarlet torrent which soaked the front of his gown. The registrar continued sucking. Sister quietly packed large swabs either side of the girl's abdomen to help soak up the deluge before it hit the deck. Eyes glazed as he felt around the hidden depths of the left upper abdomen, Hawes formed a mental image of what his experienced fingertips conveyed. He moved his hand to the right lower quadrant and his gaze snapped back into focus. By lifting with his right hand and pulling open the incision with his left, he delivered the lower part of the spleen into plain sight. It lay on the bloodied drapes, the tip reaching as far as the girl's right groin; half a burgundy-coloured rugby ball. But the real trouble lay with the upper half, still inside. Thirty more seconds.

The difficulty in removing any organ is getting at its plumbing. You can't simply rip a heating radiator or something more complex, such as a boiler, from a wall. The water pipes and any other supply (gas, oil, electricity) need to be safely cut off and all supporting attachments unscrewed or released. Foolhardy DIY extraction of such an appliance is potentially dangerous. Foolhardy extraction of an organ is deadly.

The spleen, as mentioned earlier, is stuffed behind the colon and stomach with the left kidney beneath. The plumbing – the artery and vein – is also hidden, in this case behind the pancreas. So, to access those vessels from the front – the anterior approach – requires careful and lengthy dissection of the colon, stomach and pancreas. Removing the spleen, splenectomy, is occasionally done via the anterior approach if it's exceptionally large and difficult to manoeuvre, but generally, getting at the plumbing in this way is best avoided, because the pancreas is a completely unforgiving bastard. If damaged, it will leak digestive enzymes into the abdominal cavity, where those same complex chemicals mindlessly perform the task they normally and quite safely do on protein, fat and carbohydrate (food) passing through the gut. That is, they'll digest your insides. As you might imagine, this is a prolonged, painful, and ultimately lethal process. To avoid such unpleasantness, the posterior approach has much to commend it, particularly when the splenectomy needs to be accomplished with some urgency.

Hawes directed his words to Dr Kirkby at the head of the table. He spoke loudly to pitch his voice over the incessant hissing gurgling sucker the registrar still wielded, but we were all meant to hear. 'Anna, the spleen's fractured at the back, but it's so big I'll never get it out through this hole. How's she doing?'

'Still with us,' Kirkby twanged, 'But she's still losing blood.'

'Yeah, I know. Gimme ten minutes, max.' Then he turned to the sister, 'Diathermy needle.'

He slid his left hand, palm upwards, into the left side of abdomen, lifting the muscle and skin away from the hidden deeper half of the spleen. A diathermy needle is just that: a needle with a pen-like handle attached by an insulated cable to a machine the size of a domestic fridge. He put the needle to the skin and pressed the pedal with his foot. The machine let out a continuous warning buzz, simultaneously passing a high frequency electric current to the needle tip. With heat so intense and localised it vaporises tissue, he drew the needle towards him, producing wisps of steam and smoke, along with the familiar sickly sweet stench of burnt flesh. The cut was clean, quick and bloodless, done with the effortless certainty of a correct decision made. Hawes continued through the various layers of muscle until his left hand reappeared. Within a minute, the original top to bottom incision was now joined by a horizontal one across the left upper quadrant.

'Deaver retractor,' Hawes spoke quietly, unhurried, though the dark stain of sweat on the brow of his theatre cap betrayed an inner tension. The scrub nurse, ahead of the game, handed it to him blade first. Fashioned from stainless steel and a foot long, the gently curved blade was rounded at the tip, four inches wide, with a stout handle set at a right angle. He slid the instrument into the wound, simultaneously presenting the handle to the registrar opposite, 'Pull.' The large incision gaped even wider as the retractor lifted the ribcage forwards and sideways. The spleen filled most of the abdomen. It was huge. Hawes paused for a split second, took a deep breath and exhaled slowly, letting his hunched shoulders relax. 'Now then, Mary …' for the first time he spoke to the sister by name, 'I'll probably need some help from you to lift it toward me, so give me a big swab and the long scissors, and if needs be, I'll tell you what to do, and when.'

Undaunted, she slapped the handle of the scissors into his right palm and placed the folded white swab, the size of a tea towel, into his left, leaving her own hands free to assist. 'I'm ready when you are.' For a scrub nurse, it's all part of the job.

The posterior approach to the spleen's plumbing is achieved by pulling the spleen forwards and to the patient's right, thereby getting at the "clockwork" – as surgeons say – from behind. This has the added advantage of pulling the stomach, colon, and the dreaded pancreas along with it, and protecting them from injury by any sharp instruments. The left kidney is also out of harm's way, safely stuck to the back of the abdomen.

To provide better traction than his gloved and blood-slicked left hand allowed, Hawes put the swab on the upper end of the smooth, slippery spleen and dragged it towards his midriff. The lateral ligaments, little more than stretched peritoneum, gave way readily to the scissors. Mary pushed from her side of the table as Hawes pulled and cut. Inch by inch, the spleen surfaced from the deep. A jagged five-inch slash showed along its back – the fracture Hawes felt earlier – and was still gushing scarlet. He moved the swab over it to stem the blood loss and continued pulling, gently now, so as not to cause further damage: rough handling will reduce a spleen to bloody mush. A few more deft snips and he could see and feel the tortuous spring-like artery, 'Clip.' Mary quickly passed the artery forceps with one hand, the other still supporting the spleen, 'Clip,' and another. It went on for several minutes. Clip, cut, ligature. Clip, cut, ligature, until both the artery and vein were safely divided and doubly tied off. Then, Hawes let the spleen fall back into position, packed it tightly with further swabs, and took a breather. His gown was so sodden, he wouldn't have looked out of place in a slaughterhouse. Mary busied herself scooping away the blood-soaked mess of swabs, instruments and blood clots.

Hawes turned to the anaesthetist, 'Anna?'

'Hang on a mo', Richard, give us a chance.' Like a mother to an errant child, she always used his full name when stressed or irritated. The anaesthetic registrar pushed a button on the automated blood pressure monitor to override the three-minute cycle. It hissed and clicked, pumping air into the armband hidden beneath the drapes. All eyes watched the small electronic screen come to life. Still eighty over un-recordable.

'I've tied off the main supply and packed the spleen to put pressure on it.' The surgical registrar understood the implicit message, furtively sliding a hand into the wound to lean on the packs. 'She shouldn't be losing blood now.'

'Patience, Richard, patience.'

Kirkby squeezed the blood bag connected to the left arm. A few minutes passed in silence, save for the shushing sound of the ventilator, then the pressure monitor hissed into action again, ninety over fifty. Hawes needed no further encouragement. Within minutes, the final attachments to the stomach and colon were severed, then the huge spleen was heaved into a stainless-steel bucket – yes, a bucket, it was that big – and sent on its way to the path lab. The unusual abdominal incision took half an hour to close, about twice the time it took to get the spleen out. The boss and registrar spent ages on the skin sutures so the scar, once healed, would be as neat as possible. I remember thinking all that effort was rather futile. Even if she survived, the scars would be a constant source of embarrassment, no matter how perfect they were. Then, another odd notion popped into my head: she'd probably never wear a bikini.

But survive she did.

Her post-op recovery is a blank space in my memory. Try as I might, a little girl recovering from an emergency splenectomy is nowhere to be found in my ageing grey cells, but I know for certain she didn't die. It was a frenetic time in my life and training, filled from day to day with one sick patient after another, and to a certain extent it's true one never remembers the successes, only the ones you bury. No doubt, she spent a day or two in intensive care, a week or so on the kids' ward, and was followed up in the out-patient clinic. And I would have seen her every day on my ward rounds, treated her appropriately with painkillers and other interventions, but the fact is, she's not in my head. Like most extremely sick children and young adults, she would have bounced back into robust health with astonishing speed. And once started on that path, thirty-odd other patients demanded my attention, so she left no imprint. Except one.

No, it isn't the girl as such I recall, but her laboratory results. Some bright spark in the path lab, bless their cotton socks, looked at the blood smear, read the history, did a few more tests and then sent out a report to the ward. Once there, the slip of paper was added to a score of others and put into the in-tray marked "Houseman", which naturally enough, was where I found it: … *So, given the absence of any other condition wherein splenomegaly is a feature, it seems infectious mononucleosis is the cause in this case.*

In a fraction of a sentence, the path' guys pulled together all the loose strands of the girl's seemingly trivial injury, her presentation in Casualty, the monstrous spleen with massive blood loss, and the findings at surgery of a fracture rather than a sub-capsular haematoma (so much for the Casualty consultant's opinion). As I mentioned earlier, it's damnably difficult to damage a normal spleen without access to a bus or high building. But an enlarged one will grow beyond the protection of the ribcage until the only thing between it and the outside world is the abdominal wall. All of which means, unless you happen to be a body builder with magnificent washboard abs, your spleen would be vulnerable to, say, the handlebars of a bicycle.

The causes of an enlarged spleen – splenomegaly – are legion. In the tropics, splenomegaly is widely endemic, thanks to malaria and an impressive number of other parasitic infestations, the names and lifecycles of which give medical students nightmares and more senior doctors the sense to do an internet search. The spleen, to reiterate, works as a filter. If your blood is full of nasty creepy-crawly things that shouldn't be there, it will trap and eliminate them. In simple terms, the harder it needs to work the bigger it gets. Huge spleens were once so common in tropical countries that an assassin in a crowded marketplace could reliably do his work en passant with a sharp prod to the left upper abdomen. Not as immediate as a silenced handgun or knife, but equally terminal, with the added advantage of no incriminating holes.

In the developed world, big spleens are more likely to be associated with diseases such as leukaemia, Hodgkin's lymphoma and viral infections. Of the latter, infectious mononucleosis, as suggested in the path report of the young girl, is a prime and common example. Otherwise known as Glandular Fever, or Mono in the USA, it is transmitted in saliva and for obvious reasons is also called the Kissing

Disease, though youngsters most likely catch it from shared utensils and toothbrushes. A striking feature is enlarged lymph nodes or glands (hence, Glandular Fever) in the neck, armpits and elsewhere, along with characteristic white cells called mononucleocytes (hence, Mono) seen in the blood under a microscope. You've probably had it yourself, either as a child, at which age it produces few or no symptoms, or as a young adult, when it's wretched.

I contracted it towards the end of my first year in medical school, but since the incubation period is six weeks, I've no idea who the vector was, though I'm quite certain she wasn't a bloke. I'm about to go off-piste here, but stay with me, it's vaguely amusing.

The rules dictated that "first years" must live in the Halls of Residence, where the matronly warden could oversee her charges and thereby sooth any anxiety regarding homesickness or inability to cope without mother. She conducted pre-term tours of the bedrooms, the TV lounge, restaurant, launderette, music room, gym, squash courts and other facilities. If you're the parent of a university student or a graduate yourself, you'll have been there. The bar was always studiously omitted from the schedule. In reality, of course, seventy eighteen-year-olds, each with their own single room, took to the hedonism of university life like ducks to water, and the student bar was the village pond. One of those ducks must have been the carrier who infected me.

To say I retired to my bed when I felt ill would be a gross

understatement; I simply couldn't get out of it. I awoke one morning feeling, as my mother used to say, like death warmed up: shivery, feverish and pole-axed, with the sheets soaked in sweat. Not a normal hangover then. An overwhelming weakness kept me in bed for two or three days. In the following week, I managed to get to a few lectures but gave up because the effort left me drained and drenched in perspiration. After ten days of failure to appear in the bar every evening and my insistence it was "just the flu", concerned neighbours and friends dragged my listless body to the campus GP who did an examination and took a blood sample: 'I don't think it's anything serious, but better safe than sorry.'

Mid-afternoon the next day, I was in bed and still feeling ghastly when a couple of mates came to visit. They looked decidedly shifty. 'There's a big notice on the board asking you to go and see the Professor of Haematology. It says urgent.' Although my colleagues didn't verbalise their thoughts, we all reached the same conclusion: I obviously had acute leukaemia and the Prof needed to break the bad news.

As it turned out, when I arrived in the haematology department, accompanied by one of my drinking/soccer chums, the professor wasn't there, though he'd left instructions with his registrar, a jolly-hockey-sticks type with sturdy thighs and a voice like fingernails on a blackboard, who oozed inexperience from every pore. We were standing in the middle of the lab, microscopes and technicians everywhere, and she didn't introduce herself.

'Ah, yes, thanks for coming, I've been expecting you.' The badge on the lapel of her white coat read: Haem Reg. It was too small to hold the full title.

'Why am I here?' Anxiety had me impatient for answers.

'Don't you know?' She gulped hard, clearly alarmed.

'No.'

'Are you sure? The Prof sent you a message, didn't he?'

'Yes, I'm sure I don't know. And yes, he did. The message said to come here and see him. So here I am, but it seems he's not.' The sarcasm went into orbit, way over her head.

'No, he's in a Dean's meeting ...' she noticed my shoulders and head droop at the news, '... but I'm sure I can sort things out.'

I lifted my eyes to hers in a pleading fashion, though she probably took it as menacing. 'I hope you can, I really don't feel very well.'

'Oh, er ... yes ... sorry about that. No, I don't suppose you do. So, okay, where to start? Yes, I know. You went to the student health clinic yesterday?' Eager to get something right, her head was nodding like a dashboard ornament over cobblestones. In return, I nodded once. 'Well, we've looked at it ... and it's fantastic!' With an air of finality and looking ever so pleased with herself, she smiled broadly, as if waiting for applause.

Putting a hand on a nearby lab bench to support my aching body, I glanced at my beer buddy. The twenty-minute walk to get there had exhausted me, yet with what little strength remained, I could have happily strangled the woman. He recognised my mood and quickly intervened, 'Looked at what? And what do you mean by fantastic?'

'Your blood film, of course!' She was gushing at me, even though my lips never moved. My blank face produced a further torrent. 'Ah … yes … no … I'm not explaining things clearly, am I? You see, we've got finals coming up in a few weeks and the Prof wondered if you'd be kind enough to give us some more of your blood so we can make up enough microscope slides to use in the exam. He said he's never seen such a good example of mononucleosis and I personally think your white cells are absolutely fabulous. But we need the sample as soon as possible before you get better and they all disappear. Would that be okay?' Her chest heaved, breathless with excited anticipation.

'It's Glandular Fever then,' I whispered, unsure of what she'd said.

'Yes, of course it is. Hasn't the GP told you yet?'

'No. He said it'd be a few days before he gets the results.'

'Cripes. What did you think you were here for then?'

'No idea,' I lied. 'Where do you want to take this blood?'

She finally sat me down and extracted, in Tony Hancock's words, very nearly an armful. Afterwards, my mate insisted we drop into the student bar to celebrate my not-too-imminent demise. After just half a pint, I was completely sozzled. Glandular fever, I later learned, also affects the ability of the liver to cope with alcohol. We told the final year students what to expect in the haematology exam, and oddly enough, four years down the line, infectious mononucleosis came up again. I was looking down the microscope at what was probably my own blood.

⎯⎯⎯⎯⎯⎯

Thirty-odd years passed. I'd been a consultant for twenty of them and was in my weekly evening clinic at the local private hospital. A woman of around forty came in accompanied by her husband, referred to me with varicose veins. Mundane stuff, but for a vascular surgeon with a private practice, treating women with medical insurance and varicose veins is bread and butter work. It helps with the mortgage and school fees, is generally risk free, and the patients are nearly always delighted with the results. After taking a history – fit, three children, no previous illnesses, no on-going conditions, no operations, allergies or medication – I went on to examine her, designer jeans and shoes off. To see varicose veins clearly, patients need to be on their feet, so the veins fill with blood and stand out. They were minor and could be cleared easily with injections. I was about to get up from my crouching position when I noticed a tiny surgical scar on her right ankle.

Now, surgeons are good at scars. And no, I don't mean inflicting them. Surgeons make incisions, accidents with chainsaws make wounds, excessive heat or chemicals cause a burn. Healing of such injuries always leaves a telltale scar. Most sensible adults can tell the difference between a healed burn, the neat white line of a surgical incision or a nasty ragged chainsaw scar, and a surgeon certainly would. But to a surgeon a surgical scar also opens a whole panorama of understanding: the initial illness, the symptoms, the type of operation, any post-operative infection, and much more. Surgeons will recognise their own work simply from the scar, its precise placement, the length, a slight bend here or there. Or even the work of others, "No it's not one of mine, but Joe Bloggs always curves the top end like that, I reckon it's one of his."

For a moment, I stared at the scar on the woman's ankle and quietly considered all the possibilities. There weren't any. It was from a cut-down to get at the saphenous vein.

'What's that?' I pointed.

She peered down at her foot, 'What?'

'That.' I traced my fingernail along the short white line, 'How did you get it?'

'I don't know … it's always been there. What is it?'

It's not uncommon to come across an adult who's needed surgery in childhood and subsequently grows up without any recognition of the fact it's unusual. Maybe they simply have no memory of the operation or somehow presume scars are normal. Or possibly, the scars become an integral part of their body image and no more relevant than say, the colour of their eyes or hair.

'Show him your tummy, darling,' the husband intervened.

I stood up, my knees complaining with a loud crack or two. 'You told me earlier you'd never had an operation,' a gentle admonishment, said with a smile and a sigh.

'Sorry, I forgot about it. How silly of me. But it's all so long ago …'

'No matter.' I gestured at her belly and then the couch, 'Do you mind if I have a look? It could be important.'

She lay down and I covered her bare legs with a blanket for the sake of her modesty and my decorum. Then, she pulled her jumper up to her bra.

And yes folks, there it was. The scar of the incisions I'd seen thirty-years previously: a full-length midline adjoining a left upper transverse. And let's not forget the one at the ankle, the right ankle, the one which initially at least, brought her back from the dead. It must be her. Female, white, English, and the correct age. Nobody else on Earth could fit the description and bear those same stigmata. *Could they?* Yet, if it *was* her, she was a long way from home. My surgical houseman job had been in Yorkshire.

'This probably sounds like a really crazy question, but did you happen to grow up in Harrowgate?'

She gave me a curious lopsided smile, the sort usually reserved for magicians, mind readers and unbelievable coincidences. 'Just outside, in a little village nobody's ever heard of. How did you know that? We moved down here when I was still a girl.'

'Was that before or after your operation? Bear with me, I'll tell you everything when I'm sure.'

'It must have been after. I remember starting secondary school from our new house, so I would have been eleven.'

My heart skipped a beat or three. 'Let me just finish examining you, then we'll talk.'

Out of habit I briefly palpated her abdomen, touched

the scar with my fingertips, smiled in recognition of an old friend. And remembered it all.

Sparkling technicolor images crashed through my mind, an explosion of foaming memory bubbles crowding my brain, instantly taking me back to the last century, to a happier, younger, brighter time, when every experience was chrome-shiny new, and I was fresh, keen and green. There was sadness there as well, lots of it. Sadness for that long-gone ignorant youth, a foreign stranger from someone else's lifetime, now usurped by a gnarled seen-it-all-done-it-all old man with creaky knees. Sadness too for Dick Hawes the surgeon, Anna Kirkby the anaesthetist, the Casualty consultant, the scrub nurse – probably all dead – and forgotten, by me at least. Yet here was the result of their work on that sweltering summer morning, aeons ago. And regret. Regret I couldn't tell them about it, shake them by the shoulders, leap up and down and shout, 'Hey, remember that skinny tomboy? The one with the huge spleen? Well, she's turned into a vibrant, intelligent, glowing, beautiful woman, a lover who's loved in return, a wife, and a mother of three kids. All your sweat and skill were worth it. Just look at her now. *She's absolutely ... bloody ... brilliant.*'

Only seconds passed, but when I looked up from those scars to peer into her quizzical eyes, it was as if a fuse inside me had been lit, one that burned and fizzled its way back through time itself. And then the beaming idiot grin of a young houseman who was hooked on surgery greeted her once more.

'Hello … again. You're not going to believe this, but we've met before … a very long time ago. Get yourself dressed and we'll have a chat.'

Did I ask if she ever wore a bikini? Sorry, but I would never betray a patient's confidence.

3

CLOSE SHAVES AND CASUALTY

After a year of medical and surgical houseman jobs which accustomed me to on-call bedrooms with a rostered 24/7 responsibility for a mixed bunch of in-patients, I was now a Casualty senior house officer (SHO), and one quarter of a shift system that allowed me to walk clean away at the end of each duty period. Every patient seen and treated was either discharged or admitted, but after that, there was no further role for me to play. No more thinking, planning, checking, worrying, chasing results, preparing for the boss's ward round and pondering the "what ifs" of every case. All that hassle now belonged to someone else. Until the next shift began, my mind was a patient-free zone. But I hated it. I missed the continuity of care, the closeness of daily contact with the same patients, with me seeing them improve when I'd made the right call, or intervening if I was wrong. Casualty doctoring was like eating the starter of a lavish banquet, then being denied the rest of the meal.

The job was at my alma mater, The Middlesex Hospital in Mortimer Street. Long gone now, it was the most central hospital in London, being a slow ten-minute stroll north from Oxford Street. Ten more minutes would take you across Tottenham Court Road to University College Hospital, and ten minutes in a black cab would have you at any of half a dozen other teaching hospitals, all of which boasted a Casualty unit. It's no wonder the provision of healthcare in London underwent a radical reconfiguration in the final years of the last century, though to be fair, each hospital provided first-class treatment centres for complex medical and surgical problems referred from outside the capital, and those that remain still do.

Given the surplus of Casualty units, the paucity of local residents, the huge weekday influx of office-job workers and streets grid-locked with traffic, the walk-in customers at The Middlesex were never going to attract a young surgeon intent on learning how to treat severe trauma. Indeed, Casualty was little more than a drop-in GP clinic for commuters, coupled with a minor injury unit. And at weekends it was practically dead. Management knew this, which was why the job for would-be surgeons was linked to an anatomy demonstrator position, and for would-be physicians, a medical SHO post. By dangling the appropriate carrot, they filled the vacancies, but the prize came six months later. You had to endure the tedium of Casualty first.

Oxford Street, teeming with drug dealers and blessed with hundreds of warm street-level air conditioning vents, was a magnet for victims of drug dependency and homeless persons. Consequently, they were our most frequent flyers, though at the time – towards the back end of 1976 and long before political correctness went mad – we called them junkies and tramps.

There was a junkie room carpeted with plastic-coated mattresses (easier to hose down and clean) in which those who had overdosed – OD'd – were laid in the recovery position until they regained consciousness. Being already on the soft floor, deep within the comforting grip of drugs and gravity, they couldn't hurt themselves by falling off a trolley while on a bad trip. About twelve-foot square with white-tiled walls and floor, it was probably a converted toilet or minor surgery area. At first, I thought it an inhumane way to accommodate any patient, but quickly realised it was an elegantly practical solution for a huge problem. Each morning, the room would be thoroughly cleaned of the detritus, stale odours and occasional vomit of yesterday's occupants, and all the mattresses replaced by clean ones. The next tranche of customers would then begin arriving late afternoon and early evening.

Most of the junkies were on first-name terms with the nurses who, on their knees, dutifully carried out regular pulse, respiration and blood pressure monitoring on the dozen or so bodies the room could hold. If the observations began to deteriorate, we would inject naloxone to reverse the presumed opiate (heroin, morphine, pethidine, methadone) agent. The system worked well until one rather clean and smartly dressed man, who was incorrectly assumed to be junkie, refused to stir after a few hours. The SHO on duty had the good sense to check the unconscious man's blood sugar on a finger-prick blood test and found it low. Intravenous glucose woke him in seconds. He was a diabetic, without a MedicAlert necklace or bracelet, who'd pushed too much insulin or not eaten enough carbohydrate. Thereafter, a blood glucose test was mandated for all unconscious occupants.

Unlike the junkies who were delivered by ambulance, the tramps usually walked in with minor complaints, particularly when the weather was cold or wet. This implied their normal sleeping place alongside a warm air vent was already occupied, or the charity night shelter was full. After examining the blister on a heel or toe, the grazed knee, the sore eye, we'd treat it, give them tea and toast from the staff restroom, and put them up for the night on a trolley shielded with curtains. By early morning they'd be gone, back onto the streets. The majority were alcoholics or suffering mental health issues, but their stoic courage and proud independence impressed me. Offered the plethora of social care information leaflets, they gratefully accepted the thickest ones and used them to line their shoes.

In mid-December of that year, Johnny Mathis was climbing the charts just in time for Christmas with *When a Child Is Born*, and in keeping with long-held NHS tradition, the receptionists at the front desk had decorated their small domain with ancient tinsel and fresh cotton-wool "snow" purloined from wound dressing packs. An ambulance, the white old-fashioned type with a silver bell, brought in a tramp we'd not seen before. He'd been found at the back of

Selfridges that morning, sheltering under a pile of cardboard. Barely rousable, with a thick six-month beard and dark long hair under a green woollen cap, he wore a thick greatcoat and good quality heavy boots which appeared to have come from an Army & Navy surplus store, indicating he could normally look after himself very well. The ambulance crew made the diagnosis: 'He stinks of alcohol, Doc, but the main problem is hypothermia. The best oral temperature we can get is thirty-three. We found an empty bottle of vodka nearby, so we reckon he was on a bender last night, passed out dead drunk and got cold. There was frost on his coat and beard when we picked him up. Otherwise, he seems okay. No head injury we can find, no junkie injection marks, no other injuries, no identification and no money. Oh yeah, one more thing. Under all that fuzz he looks younger than our usual clientele. No grey hair, 'bout thirty-five we reckon. And he's clean apart from superficial dirt. We don't think he's a tramp. Possibly a tourist who's been robbed as he slept it off. It's anybody's guess.'

Booze and cold don't mix well. Alcohol relaxes and dilates skin blood vessels, giving that familiar warm radiant glow. Ordinarily, shedding your body heat in such a fashion wouldn't matter much in a friendly environment, but being unconscious on a concrete pavement at an ambient night temperature below zero, as the young mystery tramp had been, will simply suck the life out of you. Another problem is that cold itself directly causes skin blood vessels to dilate;

check out your hands, nose and cheeks next time you have a snowball fight, sober or not. That bright red colour is caused by the tiny muscles controlling skin arterioles being paralysed by cold, so in effect, cold skin blushes. Furthermore, cold tissues can't extract oxygen from the blood, so it stays oxygenated and bright red. Similarly, the nerves, deprived of warmth and oxygen won't work, so your fingers and toes go numb and stiff. Once back indoors and your hands and face warm up, you'll notice a blue tinge as the blood releases its oxygen, and then white as the blood vessels constrict to stop heat escaping. Finally, as the nerves come back to life, sensation returns, and everything becomes its normal muted pink again. Incidentally, the capacity for nerves to stop working when cooled is used widely for minor interventions. A cube of ice or a spray of ethyl chloride to the skin will numb it long enough for a biopsy, blood sample or stitch without complaint, especially in a child.

If you can't escape the cold due to whatever circumstance, you'll start to shiver, which warms you in much the same way as exercise does. All that muscle contraction depends on biochemical reactions that generate heat as a by-product. The shivering response to cold is initiated by a thermostat located in the primitive brain stem when your "core" temperature drops a smidge below its normal 37C. "Core" is a notional term for the innermost part of the body, but since we're not spherical and don't have a true core, in this context it refers to the temperature of deeper organs such as the liver, heart and brain. Because the thermostat is located in the brain, short of drilling holes in the skull, the best approximation to brain temperature is reached by taking readings from the mouth or ear. If the core temperature drops below 35C, the shivering reflex stops.

Human cellular biochemistry has evolved over millennia to work best at 37C. Below this temperature, the normal chemical reactions of everyday metabolism, nerve conduction and muscle contraction slow down or stop working. Once the biochemistry starts slowing down, less and less internal heat is produced, and we get inexorably colder. A snowball-frozen hand is child's play compared to core temperature loss.

The tramp was comatose drunk. Alcohol-induced skin blood vessel dilation caused heat loss. His skin was cold due to the freezing air and ground temperature, more dilation, more heat loss. He probably shivered for a while, though the alcohol may have dampened that reflex. Either way, once his brain temperature fell to 35C, the shivering stopped, and his fate was sealed.

Treating even mild hypothermia is surprisingly difficult. Warming the body needs be done slowly and gently. The intuitive hot bath, for example, is more likely to cause circulatory collapse and death rather than recovery. A cold heart is apt to stop beating regularly, squirm uselessly (fibrillate) and won't respond to defibrillation (zapping it with electricity). Why would it? It's cold, not short of volts. And a cold brain, if it does anything at all, does stupid things like telling you to lay down in the nice warm snow. Much of what we know regarding hypothermia and its treatment has been gleaned from vile Nazi concentration camp "medical" experiments, which found the most successful therapy was to put the naked victim into a bed with two healthy, and therefore warm, naked prisoners on either side.

Since there was a prevailing shortage of warm healthy naked volunteers, what I did with our tramp was to gently undress him, attach an ECG monitor, insert a rectal temperature probe (it read 33.5C), bury him under warm dry blankets, stuck an oxygen mask on his face, and surrounded him with every mobile examination lamp I could find in the department, all proper filament bulbs that kicked out plenty of heat. Then, I took some baseline blood tests, started a slow IV line for access if it were needed, parked him in a prominent position with the curtains open so we could all keep an eye him, put a nurse on his case, and carried on seeing other patients. With Christmas approaching, his appearance generated some comments which initially were lost on me: "All we need now is Mary and Joseph." "Can't someone dangle a silver star over his head?" When I asked what all the fuss was about, I was told to take another look at my work. With his beard and long hair, and surrounded by a halo of lights, he resembled the centrepiece of a bizarre adult Nativity scene.

Before finishing my shift, his temperature had reached 35C without any untoward cardiac events and he was starting to talk incoherently in a language nobody recognised, possibly Russian. The projected line on his temperature chart indicated it would be several hours before he was up to speed, and I still had no idea what his kidneys were doing because I thought insertion of a bladder catheter would be too risky for his precarious cardiac status. So, I rang the duty medical registrar, explained the situation, had the guy admitted to a ward for the night – together with the lamps – and went home. I never did find out what happened to him subsequently, or his story. Frustrating, isn't it? As I said earlier, Casualty only ever provides the first course.

The worst thing you can do as a doctor is to get it wrong. Obviously, it's bad for the patient, but can be equally devastating for the doctor. I've seen perfectly good medics lose their nerve and give up when faced with such adversity. The trick is to have one's antennae well-tuned, especially in Casualty when anything can turn around and bite you on the arse. The moral is, when something doesn't feel or smell right, trust in intuition. Here's a few "but for the grace of" Casualty tales.

Sunday morning, just before eight. I arrived in the department to take over from the night-shift guy and met him in the coffee room for a handover. He'd had a quiet night and apart from a couple of OD's in the junkie room, there was nothing hanging around. After putting on a white coat I headed off to check on the junkies, which involved no more than peering into the room through the wide safety-glass window. They were regulars, both awake, sitting on a mattress with backs against the wall, drinking sugary lukewarm tea from large plastic beakers held in shaky hands – hot drinks were deemed a scalding hazard. Within the hour, they'd be on Oxford Street looking for another fix, and back here sometime this evening.

Somewhere behind me, I overheard a triage nurse berating some poor sod in one of the curtained sit-down cubicles. Whoever it was, she was really having a go. Mercifully, the rest of the department was deserted: 'What do you think this place is? Turning up here with a hangover … demanding paracetamol … buy it in a shop …' The verbal attack seemed so over the top and unprofessional I assumed it was aimed at one of the staff who'd arrived "unfit to work", or possibly a tramp who was trying to blag some breakfast. Either way, the nurse was behaving so abominably, I decided to intervene. Also, feeling a bit delicate myself after the excesses of Saturday night, I felt some empathy with the object of her ire. Behind the curtain, I found a staff nurse who should have known better, but didn't, and sitting in the plastic chair was a bloke about my age in jeans and a tee shirt. He looked frightened, pale and ill. I scowled at the nurse and told her to leave.

Gently, I introduced myself before starting off the conversation with something that niggled me. 'When I get a bad hangover, I have to stay in bed until at least midday or later. It's not an option. I just can't face the day and have to sleep it off.'

He spoke softly, without force or gesticulation, and his head was quite still, almost stiff. 'Same with me, but this ain't a hangover. I hardly drank anything last night and woke up with a splitting headache like you wouldn't believe, and I feel like shit. Something's not right.'

'I'm sorry about the nurse's behaviour.' He didn't reply,

or even shrug his shoulders. I pulled the curtain open and pointed, 'Look, I'd like to examine you properly. Can you make it across the room to that trolley opposite? I need you to lie down.'

He slowly rose to his feet and shuffled the ten yards like a toy robot. At the trolley, he laid himself face down, then log-rolled onto his back. It was painful to watch, and I had absolutely no idea what, if anything, was going on. After checking his pulse and blood pressure, I asked a few basic questions: he was doing a PhD at University College, lived in shared digs nearby, smoked some dope but no hard stuff, otherwise fit until now. Before examining him, I reached to the wall and flicked on the overhead light to get a better view. Screwing his eyes tight, he grunted, 'Turn it off, TURN IT OFF!'

It was, quite literally, a light bulb moment. The light hurt his eyes, so he didn't like it – photophobia. Five minutes later, I was talking to the on-call medical reg' over the phone. He sounded grumpy, as if he'd only just got to bed and was trying to catch up on lost sleep. 'I've got a guy of twenty-three here with meningitis.'

'Piss off. This time on a Sunday morning? You're fucking joking.'

'Headache, photophobia, neck stiff as a crowbar, can't straight leg raise. He's got the lot, apart from a rash, so it could be viral. It's no joke, so get down here now.'

I'd learned to be forceful with registrars, the rank immediately above me. Start a referral with, "I think I have a patient who might need ..." and they'll berate you as an indecisive idiot, resulting in a lengthy wait before you see them. Tell them exactly what's wrong, say why they're needed and how urgently, and they don't mess you about. Ever. Sure enough, within half an hour he'd seen the patient, agreed with the diagnosis, whisked him off to an isolation unit for an urgent spinal tap, and as usual, I never learned the outcome. Though I did learn something. That morning, I could have sided with the triage nurse and not intervened. But I didn't because firstly, personal experience told me a hangover victim would never go to Casualty under their own steam that early in the day. And second, putting on the overhead light was pure luck, but I've done it ever since. The nurse? She was riddled with guilt and remorse. Another lesson learned.

The next one, strangely enough, happened on the same Sunday. My shift that day was 8 a.m. to 6 p.m. For the first four hours I was on my own, but at midday another SHO started and worked till 8 p.m. before handing over to the night guy. The weekend system worked because the mornings and nights were quiet, whereas the afternoons and early evenings were relatively busy. After the meningitis patient was admitted, I saw a slow succession of simple stuff, punctuated by one old chap with a heart attack complicated by a leaking mitral heart valve. When I listened in, he had what's called a seagull murmur – cooaw, cooaw, like a seagull – and pulmonary oedema. That same medical registrar arrived in a flash.

Just before midday my colleague dutifully arrived on

time, boiled the kettle to make us coffee, and give me a ten-minute break. We chatted about the meningitis patient and the seagull murmur, both of which made him green with envy. Like most career physicians, he loathed anything to do with surgery, blood, pus, or other bodily fluids, but could be moved to ecstasy by rare medical conditions. It's in the makeup of our characters – physicians are cerebral and like solving problems; surgeons are practical and prefer to fix them. The American medical drama *House* exemplifies an extreme example.

In the pocket of my white coat were two brown casualty cards from the on-duty sister, each with a brief outline of the patients waiting to be seen. Finishing the coffee with a couple of hurried gulps, I took them out. It was time to get back to work. 'One's a …' glancing at the card, 'sprained ankle. The other's a … kid with a headache. Take your pick.'

'I'll take the kid,' he said, instantly grabbing the card from my hand. As I knew he would.

Twenty minutes later, I was hanging around the unit waiting for an ankle X-ray film to be developed and returned, along with my wheelchair-bound patient. The film was probably unnecessary, but there were standing orders to get one on all sprained ankles – missed fractures, even inconsequential tiny ones, produce litigation. Meanwhile, my oppo had seen the child and was now on a wall-mounted phone speaking to someone. Idle curiosity forced me to eavesdrop. What I heard made my jaw drop.

'… papilloedema with bitemporal hemianopia. At his age it's probably a craniopharyngioma, but he needs admitting because of the raised intracranial pressure ... Okay, I'll send him along via X-ray. By the way, his parents are with him, but I haven't told them anything yet ... Yeah, alright, I'll leave it to you. Cheers.'

Quite simply, he'd just made the most outstanding clinical diagnosis I'd ever heard. After he dispatched the family to get a skull film on their way to the paediatric ward, I tackled him about it. 'Bloody hell, that was shit hot stuff. Craniopharyngioma? Go on, admit it, you ate three Weetabix for breakfast, didn't you?'

He briefly hunched his shoulders and gave me a self-effacing smile. 'I hope I'm wrong, but I don't think so. He looks ill and the headache's been going on for weeks, worse in the morning and when he coughs. The optic discs are swollen, and he has tunnel vision. I suppose it could be a pituitary tumour, but it amounts to the same thing. There's something going on in that area and aged six it's most likely a craniopharyngioma. You know that.'

'Yeah, but I'm glad you saw him and not me. I'd probably have given him paracetamol syrup and sent him home.'

'No, you wouldn't. He's been on it for weeks and it made no difference. It was that and the history which made my ears prick up. He's a bright little lad and described the symptoms well, and when he told me his eyes were "funny", I was half-way there. A full examination and ... well, you heard the rest.'

Put the tip of your index finger on the bridge of your nose and imagine pushing it horizontally into your skull. When it's sunk in about half-way, the tip will be touching your pituitary gland. It was once thought to produce nasal mucus – *pituita* is Latin for slime – but in fact, it's the central processing unit of our hormonal (endocrine) system. Directly beneath your fingertip is the uppermost reaches of the inside of your nose, and if you were to put an imaginary finger that far up one of your nostrils, its tip would also touch the pituitary. But I don't want you to do that, not because it's distasteful – it is, I've seen my children do it – but because you can't get to the optic nerves that way. So, let's return to the finger between your eyes. Directly above the pituitary, in effect laying on your fingernail, is where the two optic nerves – one from each eye – form a cross in the shape of the letter X. In the Greek alphabet, X is pronounced chi, so the optic cross is referred to as the chiasm or optic chiasma.

If the pituitary gland, or indeed your fingernail, were to grow a tumour or a craniopharyngioma, it would expand upwards between the arms of the optic chiasma, press on or invade the optic nerves on the inside of the inverted V part of the X, and in medical parlance, knock them off. The effect is like wearing horse blinkers and is called *bitemporal hemianopia:* half-blindness in both temporal fields of vision, or tunnel vision. My colleague discovered this by simply wiggling his fingers on both sides of the boy's head. The lad couldn't see the fingers until they were directly in front of him. Try it yourself whilst peering straight ahead, you can normally see just beyond 90 degrees on either side.

Using a scope to look at the back of the eye revealed swelling of the optic disc (papilloedema), a sure sign of raised intra-cranial (inside the skull) pressure – the eye being a direct and visible extension of the brain. The expanding tumour taking up limited space within the skull caused the raised pressure, which in turn produced headaches, classically worse in the morning and when coughing, because lying flat and coughing both increase the venous pressure inside the head. Watch someone having a coughing fit or doing a headstand; their neck veins stick out and their face flushes mauve. The same happens in the brain.

A craniopharyngioma is a growth (-oma) arising from the remnant of a duct which once connected the inside of your skull (cranium) to your embryonic throat (pharynx). Put the three words together and you get cranio-pharyngioma. Biologically, it's not far removed from a simple skin cyst that commonly occurs on the scalp or face, and although it's not a cancer, it behaves like one: it grows, occupies space, presses on nerves, is difficult to remove and tends to recur afterwards. So, it's not good. The incidence is about one in a million children worldwide, yet one walked into a small Casualty department in the middle of London on a Sunday morning in 1977, and was diagnosed by an inexperienced junior doctor taking a good history and doing a proper examination, coupled with a rudimentary knowledge of anatomy. Lesson learned. If you have the ears to listen, the patient will always tell you the problem. Even six-year-olds.

I was doing a slow night shift and snoozing on the coffee room couch when a nurse woke me. 'There's a mother and baby to see you. She's having trouble breast feeding.'

The clock on the wall told me it was three in the morning. Still half-asleep, I checked my watch, but it read the same. 'What? You're having me on, aren't you? There's no way I'm seeing breast feeding problems at this hour, even if I knew anything about them, which I don't. Wake me again when I'm needed.'

'They're both here and I'm not leaving until you get up to see them.' Crossing her arms over the bib of her starched white apron, she took up a "defy me if you dare" pose, standing over me and tapping her toe. I was bloody furious. Muttering all sorts of damnations, I got to my feet and followed her to the cubicle, refused to read the triage notes on the brown card she offered, and pulled the curtains aside with unnecessary forcefulness, expecting some ill-advised practical joke. But it wasn't.

She was young, perhaps twenty, with a tear-streaked face and desperate eyes. Clean and well-dressed in day clothes, this was a purposeful visit from a worried mum who'd taken the time to change, scoop up her baby and arrive. There was no anxious man in tow, but she was wearing a wedding ring, so presumably no husband available. In her embrace was a small bundle of soft white blankets with the down-covered head of a baby visible at the top of her left arm. My heart melted, along with the anger and drowsiness, to be replaced with humiliating shame. Kneeling on one knee to be at the same level, I gently asked what brought her here at such an unusual hour?

'I didn't know what to do, doctor. My husband's away

with work so I'm on my own.' She lifted the bundle towards me, 'I don't think he's feeding properly. Every time I put him to my breast, he sucks a few times and then stops. But he's always hungry and never seems to sleep.' Her tone was even and firm. 'He's my first baby, so I've never done any of this before, and I don't know if it's him or me. If you say he's fine and everything's normal, I'll just have to struggle on. But I don't think it is and I'm worried.'

I was worried too. Something she said set off alarm bells and red flashing lights in my head, but I couldn't recall why. It was important and highly significant – my memory was screaming at me – but the dots just wouldn't join up. I bided my time with a few more questions: first child, two weeks' old, born in this very hospital, dad on the North Sea oil rigs, normal pregnancy and birth, post-natal checks okay. Still nothing, memory still wailing like a banshee. Time to take a look.

I guided Mum to a trolley and asked her to lay the baby on it. With practically no experience of neonates – patients or offspring – I thought it unusually limp and quiet. Together we unfolded the blankets and then she started undoing the poppers of what many years later I would recognise as a one-piece "Babygro". As I looked on, the child's lips and face turned from pink to a startling blue, and my brain finally took a small lurch in the right direction. 'Okay, that's fine. Just pick him back up in your arms and hold him upright facing me.' I tried to sound calm, but she was far too astute.

'What's wrong?' she hissed like a snake.

'I don't know yet. But I'd like to listen to his heart. Just hold him like that ...' His lips and face were pink again, but he seemed to be breathing far too rapidly.

Putting the business end of my stethoscope on the tiny chest, I plugged in my ears and listened. Instead of the usual lub-dub of healthy valves snapping shut, his heart sounded like an ancient steam train struggling up an icy incline; shush, shooosh, shush, shooosh ... Mesmerised, I listened longer than necessary, using the short time to gather my thoughts and piece it all together. Then, it hit me: *breathless babies can't suck; it's too much effort. That's why the alarm bells rang. How the hell do I know that? When did I learn it? No idea. This kid is a "blue baby" with serious hole-in-the-heart trouble. How was it missed on the post-natal checks? No matter. Get a chest film, then throw him to paediatrics.*

'I'm afraid he has a heart murmur,' I said with due gravity, hoping my voice didn't betray the sadness I felt for her and the baby, and the disappointment it wasn't discovered sooner. 'That's why he can't feed properly.'

Mum turned so pale I grabbed a chair and sat her down before she and the baby hit the floor. Then, she spat out a stream of invectives directed at the universe, the baby's luck, his father, life in general, God, her family, hospitals, doctors, midwives ... then fell mute, tears streaming down her face. By then, the anger had returned some colour to her cheeks, and it seemed a good moment to carry on with my plan. I called for the nurse and a wheelchair, and with Mum still clutching the child upright, led all three along the corridor to the X-ray department, and parked them in the deserted waiting room.

I found the radiographer reading a magazine in her tiny office and explained the situation. 'Denise, it's a two-week old boy with some sort of right-to-left heart shunt, probably a VSD (ventriculo-septal defect), plus other malformations. When he lays flat the venous return increases, pushes blue blood from the right ventricle into the left and he changes colour in seconds. With hardly any blood going through the lungs, he's permanently breathless. I can't have him lying flat on the table while you faff about lining things up and getting the focus right.' She nodded in agreement. Much older than me – at that time I thought anyone approaching forty to be prehistoric – I knew she had children of her own and was a slick experienced professional. Radiographers are excellent at reading X-rays and this one had helped me out on numerous occasions.

'I'll put an adult plate directly onto the table rather than under it, set up the machine aimed at the whole plate, then give you the nod. We'll probably get a picture of most of him on a film that size, but as long as you position him properly flat in the middle of the plate, the chest will be all there and good enough.'

The shot took about around five seconds to do and fifteen minutes to develop – no instantaneous digital imagery in those days, or automated processors. Denise disappeared into the dark room with the plate, extracted the film and processed it by hand with a timer, developer, wash, fixer, wash, dryer. While she was doing that, I sent the nurse, Mum and baby back to Casualty, then waited in the semi-darkness of the X-ray room. Eventually, I heard the door unlock, saw the red "No Entry" light extinguish, and she walked out, the film still dripping wet in her hand, a sure sign she'd missed out the dryer because the image had an important tale to tell. 'The plan worked, it's a good view, but it looks bad.' Leading me to the nearest wall-mounted box viewer she simply plastered the wet film to the screen and flicked the switch.

It was indeed a good view, complete with the bones of my own hands holding the child's head and pelvis: bad practice on my behalf, but clumsy lead-lined leather gloves aren't designed to hold blue babies. The heart on a chest film, being far more solid than the surrounding air-filled lungs, appears white against a dark background. A normal heart is a roughly triangular white blob occupying the middle third of the chest's width. The heart I was looking at took up most of that space. It was a hugely dilated, sick sack of muscle. The X-ray could tell me no more than that. Gratifyingly, Denise agreed, and I respected her opinion.

I woke the on-call paediatric registrar and told him the story, including my suspicion of it being missed at the post-natal check, or developing since. The child was admitted straight to the NICU (neonatal intensive care unit) and that was the end of my involvement, though for once I did get some feedback when the same registrar happened to be in the department a few days later.

'How'd that baby get on?'

'Died the following day.' It was a matter-of-fact statement.

'Jeez, that was quick. Any idea what was going on with that heart?'

'Not until the post-mortem result's available.'

'Would you let me know? I'd be interested to find out the exact pathology.'

'Soon as I hear anything.'

'Great. Thanks.'

Needless to say, he never got back to me. Not his fault: that's life as a busy junior doctor, and the shift system I was on made it likely if he did try to contact me, I wasn't there.

During my six months in Casualty, there was a constant trickle of men attending with various objects attached to their appendage. Perhaps it was the proximity to Soho with its red-light district, or maybe emergency departments everywhere see similar cases, I honestly don't know. All I can say is we saw at least one a week: various tubes, milk bottles, elastic bands, plastic pipes ... anything with an appropriately sized orifice. The most common was an "Energizer Ring". When I first saw one, I thought it was the drive band from an upright Hoover vacuum cleaner, a circle of thick rounded black rubber ensnaring the root of a painfully swollen and erect penis, the owner of which – an acutely embarrassed John Smith – remained stoic despite his discomfort, and resolutely silent regarding any further personal information. One of the senior nurses, greatly more experienced in such matters, handed me a ring cutter and a tube of K-Y jelly before I disappeared through the drawn curtains. 'You'll need these,' she advised.

A ring cutter is a clever little gizmo designed to cut through soft metal and enable the removal of wedding bands, and the like, from damaged fingers when swelling or pain precludes other methods. Resembling a cheap manual can-opener, the butterfly handle turns a small coin-sized circular saw against a thin flat plate: no matter how swollen the finger, or how tight the ring, the plate will invariably slip between metal and flesh. Thereafter, the left hand squeezes the main handles to apply pressure while the right turns the butterfly-driven saw, easily slicing through soft gold or other precious metal. Usually, the ring can be prised open, but failing this, a diametrically opposite cut bisects it into two semicircles which simply fall apart. Every emergency department and most jewellers have one.

"Mr Smith" was a greying middle-aged man. He lay on the trolley wearing a jacket, shirt and tie with his trousers and underpants around his knees, eyes pinned like tacks to the ceiling and hands balled into fists at his sides. A green surgical drape covered his indignity. I explained my intentions, to which he nodded dumbly, and then, without further ado, grasped the nettle and tackled his tackle.

The purpose of all such "gadjets erotique" is to trap blood inside the engorged penis, thereby maintaining an erection. On the downside, they are effectively a tourniquet and will strangle the flow of blood if left in position too long. Continued and increasing swelling means the devices can be impossible to remove without assistance. Tubular objects, used presumably for personal gratification, generally yielded to Vaseline, K-Y, ingenuity and patience. Elastic band-type implements tended to sink into swollen flesh and needed cutting. Mr Smith's "Energiser Ring" surrendered to the ring cutter with a resounding twang followed by an audible sigh of relief as his penis deflated like a punctured balloon. Within seconds, he sprang from the trolley, pulled his pants and trousers up, drew a £5 note from his wallet (£30 in today's money) and placed it on the pillow. Then, still avoiding any eye contact and before I could object, he left without a word. Did I pocket the dough? Of course not, NHS care is free at the point of delivery, though we all had cakes and sticky buns at teatime, with a considerable donation to the biscuit fund.

A few weeks later I attended a similar case, though on that occasion the "ring" was a stainless-steel roller bearing. Two concentric mirror-bright rings glinting brilliantly under the overhead lights, separated from each other by a dozen or more exquisitely engineered frictionless rollers allowing the outer ring to spin effortlessly around the inner one, which was pierced like an axle by a blue distended penis. The bearing weighed about a kilo and was brand new, fresh from its box, no dirt or oil. The axle belonged to a guy in his mid-twenties wearing greasy overalls. I assumed he was an apprentice car mechanic but didn't bother to ask the how or the why; they were irrelevant. Short of an angle grinder or thermal lance, it wasn't coming off without surgery. I sent him on to the urologists, who no doubt deflated the problem by sucking out the trapped blood with long needles and syringes. And yes, it makes my eyes water too.

There was also a regular stream of women unable to find or

extract their tampon. Happily, the senior nurses dealt with such cases. It's a potentially serious problem that can lead to overwhelming sepsis and death, so is not, generally, an amusing subject. Nevertheless, one evening the on-duty sister fielded a phone call, passed on to her by the receptionist, from a woman who was having difficulty. Rather than ask the lady to attend, in order to save time, inconvenience and embarrassment, Sister offered to talk her through the simple retrieval process, which included removing underwear and adopting a squatting position. She readily agreed and after a few minutes of telephonic instruction and guidance reported a successful "outcome".

'I have it. Thanks ever so much for your help.'

'Good, and well done. Now, run a nice hot bath, have a long soak and a good wash.'

'I'm sorry, can't do that.'

'A shower then, with a thorough soaping down under.'

'I can't do that, either.'

'How about a bowl of soap and water, or fill up the sink and sit in it?' Sister imagined the woman must be living in a squalid bedsit. 'Surely you can manage that?'

'No, I can't.'

'Why not?'

'I'm in a public phone box on Gower Street.'

The British TV drama *Casualty* has been running thirty years or more and takes its name from a time when every major hospital had "Casualty" writ large over one of its entrances. The term is rather archaic and probably originates from the British Army Medical Corps who assemble casualty clearing stations in areas of conflict. These days, such hospital units are invariably called A&E, or simply ED, which more accurately reflects their daily function. Many are also major trauma centres with associated helipad, cardiothoracic and neurosurgery units on site. Nevertheless, the place I worked in was Casualty, so forgive my use of the word. By the way, the last time I watched *Casualty*, the sign over the doors read, "Emergency Department".

4

AN UNUSUAL DELIVERY

The out-patient sister knocked briskly and put her head around the door without waiting, 'Maternity theatres need a vascular surgeon, immediately.' She was Irish, built like a battleship, ran the department with an iron fist, took crap from no one, and we all loved her for it. It was ten in the morning, I'd been there since eight-thirty, seen about a dozen patients and there were at least a dozen more to go. Leaving now would really bugger things up.

My clinic occupied a suite of adjoining rooms. A central office with me, my secretary, a staff nurse, and an ever-present trio of medical students. On either side, was an examination room with a patient lying on a couch. The nurse's job was to keep the couches occupied with patients whilst I flitted from room to room, examining, dictating letters to the secretary, booking tests and operations, dispensing advice, criticism, encouragement, condolences, information sheets and sundry other things. Several yards further down the corridor my registrar was doing a similar job at about a tenth of my pace and from time to time would interrupt me for guidance. The medical students were there to get under my feet and ask crass questions.

I stopped mid-flit, 'Did they say why?'

'No Sir, but the girl on the phone had the fear of God in her voice, so she did.'

I left the clinic and made my way to the maternity unit. There was no choice. The first three rules of being a consultant are attend, attend, attend; in that order with no deviation. Before going, I installed the registrar behind my desk and instructed the secretary and Irish sister not to let him screw up. For years, they'd both been my rocks in a turbulent sea of ever-changing junior staff of variable experience and not-so-common sense. They knew how the firm worked, and how I worked, even down to mimicking my voice with appropriate expletives. If I made it back in time, they'd have a few important creases that needed my iron to smooth. If not, I'd sort them out that afternoon in theatres, between cases.

With a clear head and empty schedule, I negotiated my way through the underground corridors towards maternity, a standalone building at the far end of the hospital. A call to the maternity unit was a rare and unpleasant event. Ever since a small spate of headline-grabbing baby thefts from various hospitals around the country, getting into the place was like breaking into Fort Knox. Security guards, passcodes, swipe cards, CCTV and remote intercoms were in play at every door, and once inside you then needed to fend off the attack dogs, otherwise known as midwives, whose default mode for strangers was full-on aggression: everyone was a potential baby snatcher until proved otherwise. It occurred to me I didn't know the exact location of maternity theatres. No matter, I'd get directions once I broke in. My main concern was why they wanted a vascular surgeon so urgently.

Bleeding was the obvious answer. But from what and where? Vascular surgeons are called to all sorts of bleeding from the ridiculous to the insane. Surgeons generally don't like blood, or at least, unexpected bleeding, and when it happens they tend to panic. Junior and inexperienced surgeons simply don't know what to do. The answer is to press on it – all bleeding stops with enough pressure – then take a few deep breaths and work out a plan of action, even if it's simply to call for help. The only circumstances where pressure doesn't work is with large scalp wounds, which need immediate suturing with big deep stitches. And penetrating heart injuries; pressing on the heart will stop the bleeding but also stops the heart pumping. Not good.

The worst culprits are probably orthopods, who don't like to see blood in any form and use the mantra STB: Stick To Bone. With this tactic they avoid any soft tissue liable to include blood vessels, cutting down to bone in an area they know to be safe and then staying in that plane. When operating on limbs they will drain the arm or leg of blood by elevation, squeeze it dry with an elastic compression bandage, and then apply a tourniquet to stop the circulation. This works for elbows, knees, hands and feet, but only if the surgery lasts for an hour or so, thereafter the tourniquet must come off to restore the blood flow. Even with these evasive ploys, orthopods' power saws and drills have a relatively rare but uncanny habit of nicking major vessels behind the knee or deep beyond the cup of the hip joint, resulting in the cry, 'Get me a vascular surgeon.'

In recent decades, heart specialists have morphed from simple diagnosticians using a stethoscope, cardiac scanner and ECG machine – nothing sharp or dangerous there – into interventional therapists, regularly sticking all sorts of long pointy things into peripheral arteries and pushing them upwards into the heart and coronary arteries. The potential to wreak havoc at the entry/exit puncture wound or anywhere along the route is clear, and vascular surgeons working anywhere near an interventional cardiac unit get a steady stream of business from that quarter. Internal bleeding or blockage when the line perforates or damages an artery is the norm, but the most frustrating call is when the long line or tube "gets itself" knotted due to poor operator technique and stuck within a deep and not easily accessible artery or vein. No life-threatening bleed, but a major and dangerous operation on a patient with known cardiac disease, all for the sake of a knot.

Walking more briskly now, I still couldn't fathom why maternity theatres needed me. All they did there were caesarean sections and repair perineal tears and cuts. Try as I might, I couldn't foresee any need for special vascular intervention. Obstetricians are also gynaecologists – the specialty's called Obs & Gynae after all – and the only surgical emergency in obstetrics, apart from foetal distress requiring an immediate caesarean, is uncontrollable post-partum bleeding which is easily treated by hysterectomy, an operation they do for gynaecological disease every day in main theatres. Given that Obs & Gynae is a discipline whose only major operations are removal of womb (hysterectomy) and removal of foetus (caesarean section), whoever called for help must be well versed and practised in both procedures, so shouldn't have run into trouble.

Having said that, there's a general surgical aphorism that maintains gynaecologists actually do four major operations: hysterectomy, hysterectomy with damage to the right ureter, hysterectomy with damage to the left ureter, and hysterectomy with damage to both ureters. The ureter is a thin tube a few millimetres in diameter that connects the kidney in the loin to the bladder in the pelvis. Urine produced by the kidneys flows down both ureters and collects in the bladder from where it is voided at opportune moments. Through no fault of their own, the ureters on both sides happen to pass close to the right and left uterine arteries. In order to remove the uterus without a bloodbath, said arteries need to be tied and divided, and it's at this point the ureters can also be inadvertently tied, divided, or both. This is not a good thing because it does no end of harm to the patient and her kidney(s), while simultaneously ruining the gynaecologist's reputation. The one mitigating factor in such a disaster is that it wouldn't involve me, the cry for help being, 'Get me a urologist.'

I found the maternity theatres with help from a midwife who accosted me with knitted eyebrows, bared teeth and a snarl, 'Who are you and what are you doing here?' My photo ID card soothed the savage beast. 'Down to the end of the corridor, turn left and they're a few yards further on. Number One's on the right and Two is on the left.' Still in a suit and tie, I followed her directions, intending, as is usual in these situations, to put a friendly face around the theatre door to announce my arrival to the crew inside with something like, "Hi, I'm here, keep pressing on it. I'll get changed and be with you in a tick."

At the end of the passage I turned left and immediately spotted where I was needed. Blood was trickling from beneath the door of Theatre One and pooling in the corridor.

The pleasantry of putting my head around the theatre door seemed superfluous, so I went straight to the changing room. While rapidly stripping off and donning theatre greens, my mind went back to the only other occasion when I'd seen blood seeping out from under an operating theatre door. It was an all-night liver transplant in a South London teaching hospital, and I'd been pissed off because my morning list was delayed while the transplant surgeons finished off. Once changed into greens, I had a choice of footwear. Clogs or boots? Under the circumstances, I chose the white rubber boots.

Pushing open the theatre door, the first person I spotted was the anaesthetist and my heart rate went down a peg or two. He was a big bloke in every respect. British to his roots, but with an ancestry from the Far East, at school he'd gained the nickname Sumo and it stayed with him. To my eye, he resembled a Buddha rather than a wrestler, but I suppose like most of us, middle age spread added even more to his girth. Quietly spoken, wise beyond his years, an exquisitely brilliant anaesthetist, a polymath with a titanic intellect, and a chess prodigy, he gassed for one of my regular weekly operating sessions, liked a beer, adored cricket, and was a good mate. With Sumo in charge at the top end, the battle, whatever it proved to be, was half won.

When in theatres, one wears a cap and mask which hides most of the face, but accentuates our most expressive feature, the eyes. I smiled at him with a "Thank the Lord you're here," look. He nodded his head slightly, as if to say, "Likewise, thanks for coming," then tipped it sideways towards the operation and the surgeon, "Now get your arse down there and sort this bloody mess out." I knew immediately Sumo had instigated the call to get me there. I also surmised this wasn't strictly a vascular problem. There's a song about speaking without saying a word; whoever wrote it must have some operating theatre time.

Still not scrubbed, I paddled towards the operating table. Boots were definitely the right choice, though to be fair, some of the floor was dry so there was clearly a slight incline towards the door. The surgeon was the senior Obs & Gynae consultant, a decade or so older than me. Peering over his shoulder into the abdomen, I tried to sound upbeat – even though my spirit could have wept at the sight: 'Hello Steve, how can I help?' It looked like a scene from *The Texas Chain Saw Massacre*.

'This was an unexpected intra-abdominal pregnancy. I've done the section and the baby's fine, but there's a lot of bleeding.'

Then, I realised what I was looking at. All the pelvic organs were plastered with something I'd not encountered since my student days. From the bladder in front to the rectum and lower colon at the back, all were covered with placenta. He was dabbling at something in the middle.

'So, what are you doing now?'

He muttered, 'A hysterectomy.'

Incredulous, I asked, 'Why?'

But he kept his head down and gave no answer. I glanced at Sumo, then the scrub nurse. Their eyes mocked me, "We know what you're thinking."

I was thinking the man was trapped in the surgical Twilight Zone, frightened out of his wits with a brain so overloaded with anxiety it had shorted out and shut down. Compelled by the need to do something, *anything*, to salvage the situation, he'd regressed to the only action he was capable of. Namely, a hysterectomy.

Psychologists refer to the arousal/performance curve, where increasing arousal such as stress, urgency and pressure to do well heightens the quality of performance, but only up to a certain point. Thereafter, further arousal causes it to plummet as fast as a piano pushed over a cliff. It's called the Yerkes–Dodson law and is a recognised function of every human activity, from tying your shoelaces to spacewalking. The upslope of the curve is extended by experience, practice, and familiarity with the task in hand; the downslope hastened by the opposites. Steve, beyond any logical thought, was firmly clinging to that plunging piano in the vain hope it would somehow sprout wings and fly. He needed help and direction. 'Tell you what, why not put a big pack in there and press on it for five minutes while I get scrubbed, then I'll give you a hand.'

Let's pause here and consider the parasitic condition called pregnancy.

A parasite is an organism that lives in or on another organism (the host) and derives nourishment from it, usually at the host's expense. The word comes from the Greek, *parasitos*, someone eating at another's table, and yes, we've all entertained that type of dinner party guest: no wine, no flowers, no chocolates, no fun. Countless parasites afflict humans: fleas and ticks, intestinal worms, liver and lung flukes, eye worms, brain worms, protozoa, bacteria, fungi and viruses. Many have complex and obscure lifecycles involving different transitional hosts or stages, which take years of scientific research, intuition, and pure luck to unravel. One thing however is abundantly clear, successful parasites do not want to kill their host because it would be self-defeating and rapidly lead to the extinction of both species. Rather, their fervent desire is to live a long life, mature into adulthood and reproduce, thereby passing their offspring onto other hosts. Parasites need the host to stay reasonably healthy, though probably weakened, for as long as possible. A tapeworm, for example, will reside in your gut for twenty-five years or more. In the case of a human embryo, the parasitism lasts for nine months and arguably longer – let's say until financial independence. That's about the same lifespan as the tapeworm, but at least the worm won't beg you for a car when it's seventeen. The placenta deals with those first nine months.

A woman's two ovaries are quite close to the womb (uterus) and all three are nestled deep within the pelvis. By close, I mean as Birmingham (the ovary) is close to London (the uterus) when looking at the UK (the abdomen) as a whole. Every month, one or other of the two ovaries spits out a microscopic egg (ovum) into the Birmingham suburbs. The egg could theoretically end up anywhere (Cardiff, Glasgow, Aberdeen), but usually finds itself at the top of the nearest motorway (the fallopian tube, "Your tubes, madam.") and heads south to London. For the tiny ovum, this is the equivalent of you or me doing the journey on foot. During its travels, if it is to become fertilised, it meets millions of comparatively minuscule but vigorous sperm heading north, one of which penetrates the egg casing, their genetic material combines, and the beginnings of an embryo is formed.

Normally, the embryo settles in London (the uterus), puts down roots (the placenta), taps into oxygen and other nutrients, grows into a foetus, and nine months later is ready to begin the next stages of its parasitic existence: breast feeding, pocket money, private education, mortgage deposit, wedding costs, grandchild-minding, and all the rest of it. If this analogy doesn't sit easily with you, bear in mind that in order to block any detection and rejection response from the mother's immune system, the placenta produces the same defensive chemicals as parasitic intestinal worms.

And if you're still not convinced, we'll now take a closer

look at the placenta (Greek: *plakous*, flat cake). A human placenta is the size and shape of a large dinner plate and needs two cupped hands to hold. In the Western world not many mothers, and fewer fathers, have seen one, which is probably for the best, and it is never, ever, shown in TV dramas or movies with childbirth scenes. The "afterbirth", as it is also known, is delivered about twenty minutes after the main event, or rather squeezed dry and ejected by the rapidly contracting uterus. A profoundly ugly, alien-looking monster, glistening with mucus and thick fluid, with a rope-like tail of umbilical cord, it should by rights leap to the floor of the delivery room, gloop-slither-skitter into the ventilation conduits and subsequently be tackled by Sigourney Weaver (*aka Ripley*) with a flame-thrower. However, in my experience, the midwife puts it into a bowl and secretes it off to the sluice room where it lies alone, ready and waiting to pounce upon its next unwitting victim. Sorry, I was carried away there. I should have said, where it waits to go for incineration. My whimsy, however, is nothing compared to what happens in some cultures of the real world. Full burial ceremony for the dead "twin", cooked and eaten, perhaps with fava beans and a nice Chianti, burned and the ashes ingested as a contraceptive, or sold for processing by the cosmetics industry. The latter was once common, though now the monster has legal rights and the practice is generally frowned upon.

The dinner plate of placenta has two sides. The business side is lumpy, velvety, dark red and resembles the surface of a cauliflower. It is composed of microscopic fingers of blood vessels that burrow deeply into the mother's uterus and swap waste products for nutrients. The other side is where all those millions of capillaries coalesce into recognisable arteries and veins that, in turn, merge into the umbilical cord. A living (or should that be functioning?) placenta is a mass of throbbing arteries and veins, as is the pregnant uterus, transformed by placental hormones from a small nub of muscle into an elongated spheroid of pulsating fecund vascularity, or an egg casing in an *Alien* movie. If a placenta fastened itself to your back, you'd seek help, pronto, but if some kindly person attempted to peel it off, you'd probably bleed to death. On a more serious note, all that extra vascularity and the blood therein is needed to feed the rapidly growing unborn child snuggled inside the uterus. Depending on the size of the baby, a mother's blood volume increases by as much as a quarter during pregnancy and gives her that healthy radiant glow, but also puts quite a strain on her heart.

Not uncommonly, instead of London (the uterus), the embryo sets up home on the hard shoulder of the motorway (fallopian tube). The medical term for this is an ectopic pregnancy – not where it should be. A tubal pregnancy is doomed to failure because the foundations are too shallow, and potentially deadly because the placenta with its burrowing for nutrients, and the embryo growing ever larger, rupture the tube and cause catastrophic bleeding at around eight weeks or thereabouts. Many people will have experience of a relative or friend needing emergency surgery for a ruptured tubal ectopic. I certainly do, both personally and through dealing with it within the realms of "look-see" (laparotomy) general surgery.

If tubal pregnancy is relatively common, an ectopic intra-abdominal pregnancy is as rare as hen's teeth. The vast majority are probably not detected because the embryo fails to establish a sufficient blood supply, dies and is reabsorbed. Those that survive and grow usually cause mischief due to the placenta attaching itself to the gut (Cardiff), liver (Glasgow) or spleen (Aberdeen), and end up being surgically removed. An intra-abdominal pregnancy maturing to a healthy full-term delivery is as likely as rocking-horse manure.

I'd never seen one, never expected to, never studied it in depth, and presumably, neither had Steve. Yet, standing at the sink washing my hands and scrubbing my nails, I knew from first principles what was needed. And hoped I could achieve it.

Back at the table, I was gratified to see he'd followed my instructions. A pack and two fists had stemmed the bleeding to a trickle. Now that I was there, he relaxed the pressure and made to remove the big swabs. Shaking my head, I guided his fists back into position. The anaesthetist was my first concern. 'How's it going, Sumo?'

'Twenty units so far. FFP's going in. Clotting's shit. BP's stable at ninety.'

So, twenty units of blood transfused, a huge amount, getting on for ten pints. Fresh frozen plasma, full of lovely clotting factors, also going in. The lab clotting tests were bad. Blood pressure low, but not falling. All pretty much as expected. The clotting – or rather lack of it – was the biggest problem.

If you cut yourself shaving or preparing a meal, you expect to spontaneously stop bleeding within a few minutes. This happens because the wounded tissue starts a chain reaction in the blood – specifically the platelets and plasma – resulting in a whole load of clotting factors being activated in a biochemical cascade, which finally produces a blood clot. Without the wound, the blood won't clot, which is a good thing; you don't want your blood clotting for no practical reason. Without all the clotting factors, the blood won't clot, ever. Haemophilia, the curse of the Royal House of Romanov, is most often caused by an inherited absence or deficiency of Factor VIII, which gives you some idea how many of the damn things there are. When I last checked there were twenty-nine of the little beggars. In a bid for greater clarity and understanding, after discovering Factor XIII the experts stopped using Roman numerals and adopted proper names, including (I promise this is true) three called Protein Z, Protein C and Protein S. So now everything's crystal.

Bleeding excessively as a result of surgery or other trauma will eventually deplete the body's reserves of clotting factors to the point where blood no longer clots. Of course, no clot means continued bleeding, though as we say in the trade, bleeding always stops in the end. Fresh frozen plasma, harvested from donated whole blood, is in essence a broth of all known and possibly as-yet-unknown clotting factors.

And Sumo was chucking them in like a man possessed.

'Sumo, can I get cracking, or would you like some catch-up time?'

'Let me get another unit of FFP into her first. I'll tell you when.'

I crossed my arms to stop my hands wandering, knowing from hard-won vascular experience that fiddling in such circumstances disturbs the clotting process and increases the bleeding. Better to do nothing for ten minutes, allow nature to do her work and pass time with my colleague, learning about the patient. The exact details of the history Steve related are hazy because they weren't pertinent to the job in hand, and with this sort of acute problem a surgeon tends to live in the moment. It was the woman's fifth or sixth child, a good bunch in any case, and being such a seasoned veteran of pregnancy and childbirth, she'd pretty much ignored antenatal clinics and carried on regardless. Presumably, she never had a scan either. Being well past her delivery date and with no signs of going into labour, an elective C-section was scheduled for that morning.

As he droned on, I began wondering where all the blood was coming from. The placenta, cord and baby are a sealed unit containing a small but finite volume of blood. With the baby and a short length of cord gone, the placenta itself and remaining cord could only contain a minimal amount of the stuff. And it wouldn't be circulating, because the baby's heart was no longer in the equation.

The mother is also a sealed unit, but with a much larger volume of blood. The placenta doesn't suck on the mother's blood in the manner of a vampire or mosquito; rather, at a microscopic cellular level, the placenta and the mother's tissues exchange oxygen and nutrients for waste products. To enable this, the blood flow through the placenta and through the uterus is huge, but the two circulations don't mingle. If you cut the placental vessels you don't get Mum's blood, and likewise, if you cut Mum you don't get placental blood. Even if the placenta bled out, it couldn't possibly be enough to cover the floor. I then realised the scarlet liquid under my boots was probably amniotic fluid (the baby's bathwater; the "waters" which "break") mixed with a small amount of placental blood, and a whole damn lot of Mum's, together with most of the blood and FFP Sumo had already transfused into her. And of course (Ding!), for reasons unknown, amniotic fluid is as good as Russell's Pit Viper venom for really buggering up the clotting biochemistry. To reiterate, venom from a viper bite causes death by spontaneous bleeding because it poisons the clotting mechanism, and a Russell's Pit Viper is not only a big bastard, it's particularly venomous. In a test tube under laboratory conditions, human amniotic fluid, drop for drop, is up there with it. Since Mum's belly and her incision were, or had been, awash with the equivalent of viper venom, some of it surely would have seeped into her general blood circulation. Finally, I had a handle on the poor clotting results the lab reported and snapped out of my reverie. 'Steve, where do you think all this blood's coming from?'

'Dunno, it's everywhere.'

Typical response. He wasn't panicked with me there,

but twenty minutes earlier, on his own, he was blind with it. I imagine that's why he started doing a hysterectomy. If you go to a baker, he'll sell you bread. If you go to an orthopod, he'll sell you a bone operation. A neurosurgeon, and your brain gets it. An obstetrician/gynaecologist offers a caesarean or hysterectomy. This woman was getting his full repertoire. 'How far did you get with the hysterectomy?'

'The left side is tied off. The right side's still to go.'

I mentioned earlier the unfortunate tendency of gynaecologists to tie or divide ureters, so simply had to ask the vulgar question, 'Did you identify the ureter?'

'It's a sub-total, nowhere near the ureter.'

At least that was a sensible decision. By that, I mean if you're going to remove a uterus for absolutely no discernible reason, do yourself a favour and make it sub-total. A sub-total hysterectomy leaves the cervix behind and doesn't involve cutting into the vagina, a potential source of infection. It's also a quicker procedure and the ureters are generally safe. The downside is that leaving the cervix in situ opens the door to possible future cervical cancer. But she needed to live long enough for that. And right then, if I couldn't stop the bleeding, her life expectancy could be measured in minutes.

When Sumo gave us the go-ahead, Steve and I removed the packs. The view was clearer but still bloody, with constant oozing from the wound edges. Deep in the pelvis, the dome of the normal-sized non-pregnant uterus floated about in a sea of macerated placenta and blood. My brain-frazzled colleague had clearly dissected through the placenta to get at the uterus. The bleeding didn't alarm me: it was ooze and, though considerable, was controllable. The only bleeding that puts my heart rate up is from major veins, because they're tissue-paper thin, easily damaged, won't hold a stitch or clamp readily, and will bleed … and bleed … and bleed … until the patient dies.

What did exercise me, what I couldn't work out, was why there *was* so much bleeding. I examined the placenta; it covered the whole pelvis and the organs within it like a thick family-sized pizza, side to side and back to front. I could see the back edge lying over the rectum and colon and followed it forward with my fingers, over the uterus, further forward over the bladder to the pubic bone, then up the anterior abdominal wall towards the incision, until I could see my fingers once more. Quickly checking the other side of the wound … yes, there it was again … almost up to the umbilicus, more placenta but thinning out. Then, the penny finally dropped.

It was a standard Pfannenstiel incision, otherwise known as a bikini-line incision, because long ago it would be hidden beneath the waistline of bikini briefs. The incision had gone straight through the placenta, which was plastered to the inner surface of the abdominal wall. It must have bled like a stuck pig, from both the baby's side (the placenta) and the mother's (the abdominal wall). Coupled with not finding a uterus to cut through, and the amniotic sac immediately rupturing to release possibly litres of fluid, our Steve must have nearly had a heart attack. Luckily, a caesarean section, falsely attributed to the manner of Julius Caesar's birth (*see end of chapter for details*), is a bit of a smash-and-grab raid. The baby would have been out within seconds and the cord clamped, thereby saving it from too much blood loss. However, the problem with the mother's side still bleeding remained, not helped by the half-completed hysterectomy and poor clotting. The dome of the uterus had been coaxed by the placenta into massively increasing its blood supply; likewise, the abdominal wall with its surgical incision, and all the vessels were severed. The abdominal wall was no problem – like the scalp, it needed big stitches. I was still none the wiser as to why we were in the position of having to complete a half-done and needless hysterectomy, but didn't press the matter – Steve's brain was frazzled enough, without the need to add further injury. Instead, I consoled myself with, '*At least he didn't damage the colon and bladder by trying to peel the placenta off. Then, we'd literally be in the shit, and truly pissed off.*'

I put in another big pack and pressed hard on the whole lot, including the incision. Then, I explained to Steve, in a voice all could hear, what I reckoned was going on, finishing with, 'So, let's get the uterus out first and we're almost home.' In the event, the hysterectomy was straightforward. A big clamp to the dome of the uterus stopped the bleeding and worked as a handle to hoick it north, allowing access to the normal anatomy further south. A few clips and ties to the uterine vessels (I made sure the right ureter was safe, as well as double-checking the left), a knife to amputate it from the cervix, some hefty stitches to the stump, and it was out.

I put a few stitches around the hole in the middle of the placenta to slow the ooze, and put pressure on everything else by packing the pelvis and lower abdomen with about five metres of Caesar roll: nothing to do with obstetrics, it's a metre-wide thinly woven muslin which comes rolled like a bolt of cloth, and if you wore it you'd look like a Caesar in a toga. However, a good amount of it packed into a bleeding abdomen is a fair substitute for the surgeon's fists, and allows him to get on with his life, at least for a short time. Then, I began closing the incision with big nylon sutures through the whole anterior abdominal wall. It was an industrial stitch, incorporating the skin, muscle, the transected placenta and a strip of muslin, designed to strangle the possibility of any further ooze. If she survived, at the very least she'd need a change of pack and a "look-see" tomorrow, the day after that, and so on. As my hands worked, I planned her near future and realised there was no point waking her up.

'Hey, Sumo, do we have an ITU bed for this woman?'

'Yes, we do.' He was way ahead of me.

'Blimey, how'd you manage that?' An available ITU bed was a rare thing indeed.

'Remember your aneurysm from yesterday? They've kicked him out early and sent him to a ward to make room for her.'

'Bloody typical.'

For three consecutive days, I took her back to theatre to change the pack. Meanwhile, the ITU staff stabilised her clotting and blood count with more blood and FFP, kept her kidneys working, her lungs ventilated, and her skin healthy, free from bedsores. Each time I re-opened the incision, the placenta was shrinking at a remarkable rate. It had done its job for nine months and now, deprived of the baby's life-giving blood circulation, was simply dead tissue. No longer able to hide from, and defenceless against the mother's immune system, the alien interloper was overwhelmed by millions of hungry white cells, all primed for attack and hell-bent on destruction.

The last time I looked, the pizza of placenta was no more than a thin film, the ooze of blood negligible. Everything appeared pink and healthy, with no pus, no smell, no infection. Her parameters – temperature, pulse rate, haemoglobin, urine output, clotting – were fine. There seemed no good reason to continue the daily inspection of her entrails, so I took an odds-on gamble, removed the Caesar roll, sewed her up properly, layer by layer, using a neat skin suture, and told the anaesthetist, one of Sumo's underlings, to wake her up. A few days later she left ITU, went back to the maternity unit and met her baby for the first time. Within a week, they were both at home.

It was a happy ending. Especially so, because her ITU bed was vacated just in time for that day's routine aneurysm patient.

Having recounted this tale, it occurs to me some readers may wonder if the obstetrician received any form of sanction for his seemingly poor performance. The answer, quite rightly, is no, and there was never any question he should. Within the confines of such a limited specialty, he performed as well as would be expected of any other obstetrician encountering an extremely rare situation. Being highly skilled in only two major operations (caesarean section and hysterectomy), coupled with a lack of experience or practice in any other surgical discipline, dealing with such horrendous bleeding was outside his competence. Which explains the correct and timely call for help.

But the incident does raise a bigger question. Without doubt, specialists are extremely good at what they do, with statistics to prove it. Sub-specialists (or should that be supra-?) have even better figures, but within ever more narrow boundaries to their training and capabilities. That's fine if the patient has a highly specific, finely defined and accurately diagnosed problem, gets to see the correct practitioner, and the operation goes well with no unexpected findings or complications. But surgery always has the propensity to throw a curveball or googly when you least expect it, and for someone with only a hammer and a screwdriver in their toolbox, everything needs to be a nail or a screw.

Over recent years, there's been an explosion in sub-specialties. A normal orthopaedic unit, for example, is likely to have at least one hand, foot, knee, hip, elbow, shoulder, and spine specialist, and a large unit may also boast a bone tumour expert, with a few others besides, who deal with even rarer conditions. Each individual would dearly like to see nothing else, do nothing else, operate on nothing else, but their own sub-specialty patients. That would make it a nice, comfortable, nine-to-five, five-day-a-week job, with no unplanned emergencies to upset their normal schedule, disrupt a full night's sleep or interfere with every weekend off. The trouble is, in the real world, emergencies account for at least half the work of any surgical unit, and all members of the unit are signed up and paid to muck in and do them on a shared-rota system.

Let's suppose the hand surgeon suddenly and spuriously declares that since her routine job has comprised nothing but hand surgery for years, she no longer feels sufficiently practised and competent to continue being part of the emergency on-call rota for general orthopaedics. She claims to have become so de-skilled it is impossible for her to fix a broken hip say, or a fractured arm, with the required degree of expertise. Indeed, having announced her lack of ability to the world, for her to continue doing such emergency surgery would be morally, ethically and medico-legally indefensible. However, as a concession, she would be happy to help with hand injuries and would consult when asked.

Her declaration is, of course, bogus. Much like a pizza chef saying he will in future only tackle Hawaiian with pineapple topping rather than any other recipe, because that's his favourite. By discounting years of training and even more years of regular emergency surgery, equivalent to topping pizzas of every variety, she has invented a ruse to excuse herself from the onerous on-call rota.

"Hang on a minute ..." all the other experts chime, "we're in the same boat too. We'll have some of that. What, no on-call for emergencies? Yessiree, bring it on." The hip man, sadly, can't jump aboard because fractured hips are a huge part of such work. Saddled with the prospect of doing all the on-call emergencies himself, he comes up with a workable but impossibly expensive solution. "Let's advertise for at least three or four additional sub-specialists in orthopaedic emergencies, so they can do all the on-call. And while we're at it, why not get a sub-specialist orthopaedic vascular surgeon as well, to deal with all that pesky bleeding."

Of course, no such specialists exist until the advert creates a market. Then, every recently qualified junior looking for a consultant job will reinvent himself, and his CV, in order to apply.

Such shenanigans go on in many surgical units, but presently are largely resisted by strong, competent, sensitive, and careful management: "Bugger off then, you're no good to us, or go and get yourself retrained at Pizza Hut. Which do you want?"

Nevertheless, I fear the surgical sub-specialty situation may be at a tipping point and common sense will not prevail. A similar scenario played out twenty odd years ago in medical units, when many specialist physicians pulled the same stunt and were allowed to get away with it. Emergency medicine was in disarray for years.

A last word on the history and origin of caesarean section, which frankly, is as transparent as mud. Someone has probably written an entire thesis on this subject, but here is my short filtrate of the quagmire. The Oxford English

Dictionary tells us that *caesus* is the past participle of the Latin, *caedere*, "to cut". In ancient Rome, cultural taboo and the law forbade the burial of a dead pregnant woman, so the dead baby was cut from her beforehand and presumably dealt with separately. Yet many women died during childbirth, so if the cutting was done expeditiously, the baby might still be alive. Some opinion – notably, Pliny the Elder – has it that an ancestor of Julius was one such, and thereby gained the surname Caesar which was passed on to future generations. The noun Caesar eventually became synonymous with Emperor – that's why there were so many subsequent Caesars – and was also used as a verb to describe the surgical procedure. The latter form is in use worldwide, though many countries use the word Emperor. In Germany, for example, pregnant women have a Kaiser operation.

One thing, however, is abundantly clear, there is no way a live pregnant woman could ever survive such an ordeal at that time. If the operation itself didn't kill her, the bleeding and infection afterwards surely would. Since Julius Caesar's mother, Aurelia, is recorded as being fit and well during his lifetime, he could not have been delivered by C-section.

5

TRAINING TO BE A SURGEON

To surgeons of a mature age, particularly those who trained in and around London, the names David Slome and Frank Stansfield will bring a wry smile and a quotation, my own favourite being, "What is revision? Revision is learning for the first time on the night before the exam." Yes, perhaps you've already guessed, less than two years after passing Finals, I was on the swotting treadmill again and faced more exams.

To become a Fellow of the Royal College of Surgeons (FRCS), I first needed to pass the Primary, or part-one examination. This is an in-depth review of the candidate's knowledge of human anatomy, physiology and a good chunk of pathology, using both written (MCQ) and live oral (viva voce) testing. The format has changed over the last twenty years, but the subject matter remains the same and the pass rate still miserable at around one in five. The main hurdle to success, as ever, is anatomy. If you're hoping to make a living from sticking sharp things into fellow human beings without killing them on a regular basis, you need to know anatomy forwards, backwards and sideways. And learning anatomy to the level required to be a surgeon, is as hard as it gets.

Pre-clinical medical undergraduates at one time did a year of anatomical dissection on preserved corpses. They were helped in this endeavour by recently qualified doctors acting as anatomy demonstrators, who accepted the job and feeble pay in order to spend six months absorbing enough anatomy to pass the Primary. I was lucky enough to land such a post, and at the age of twenty-four, by always being a few pages ahead of them in the textbook, managed to fool the eighteen-year-old students into believing I knew my stuff.

Along with shedloads of Latin names, anatomy requires many lists to be committed to memory, and because the subject does not yield to logic or intuition, the use of mnemonics is rife. The anatomic variety are somewhat tasteless, usually amusing, and have been passed down over many generations. Thus, "Two Zebras Bit My Cock," tells me the order and names of the five facial nerve branches, Temporal, Zygomatic, Buccal, Mandibular and Cervical. Likewise, "Oh, Oh, Oh, To Touch And Feel A Girl's Vagina And Hymen," the twelve cranial nerves, and "As Sue Lay Flat, Oscar's Passion Slowly Mounted," the eight branches of the external carotid artery. There are many more I could spout, but most would make you blush. In addition to occupying my days with teaching risqué mnemonics and anatomy to medical students, with no clinical job and therefore no shift or on-call commitment, I was able to go to night school. It was March 1977, Queen and ABBA dominated the album charts, Fleetwood Mac's *Rumours* had just been released, and the first *Rocky* film won the Oscar for Best Picture.

The Slome-Stansfield Primary revision course ran for about thirty years and yielded a pass rate of 85%. Slome was a retired professor of physiology, Stansfield a retired anatomist, and both were renowned for being brilliant and entertaining teachers. Five nights a week, with a few Saturday mornings if it was behind schedule, the course ran for three months and finished just before the exam. Slome and Stansfield taught alternate weeks of physiology and anatomy respectively, but would occasionally swap if one had a prior engagement. It rapidly became apparent each could cover the other's subject with equal aplomb, expertise and memorable humour.

On the first evening a hundred young men (I don't recall any women) sat down in Caxton Hall, Westminster, famous at the time for being the registry office of choice for rich celebrity weddings. At the front of the hall stood Stansfield, a large imposing figure in a tailored double-breasted suit, he seemed to occupy even more space than his ample frame allowed. Alongside him was a large blackboard on an easel. And that was it. No desk, no chair, no notes, no script, not even a briefcase. He produced a stick of white chalk from his pocket, 'Gentlemen, tonight we shall cover the anatomy of the left petrous temporal bone,' and slashed a single straight line across the board. 'Draw that, and if you can't draw that, well I'm sorry, there's no hope for you.' Groans of dismay arose from the assembled crowd. If a more complex area of human anatomy exists, none of us could think of it. We were being thrown in at the deep end and some would drown. Three hours later, Stansfield put the chalk back into his pocket. 'Gentlemen, I suggest you pin the diagram you have just drawn to the wall of a small room you visit often. As the examination looms closer, you will find you go there more frequently.' Armed with pages of notes and a complex diagram concerning just one small skull bone, I found the nearest pub and downed a beer or three. I wasn't alone. By the following evening, the class had shrunk to eighty.

Slome's tutorials were equally in-depth though his style was more animated – in keeping with his slim athletic figure – with long sessions of Q&As. 'Speak up boy: if the examiners can't hear your answers, they'll fail you. Come on, stop dithering, make a decision, surgeons have to make decisions all the time …' he swished a karate chop through the air, 'AMPUTATE NOW. Even if it's wrong, MAKE A DECISION. On your gravestone I want them to write, HERE LIES A SURGEON, SELDOM CORRECT BUT NEVER IN DOUBT.'

By the end of the course, there were perhaps only fifty diehards left, but we all felt sufficiently prepared and practised, particularly those of us who'd been doing anatomy demonstrator jobs, to sail through the exam. And the handful of anatomy demonstrators, including me, helped the less fortunate by inviting them into our dissection rooms to get re-acquainted with the real – albeit pickled in formaldehyde – thing. Slome and Stansfield achieved exactly what they'd set out to do; cut out the dead wood, the "also-rans", those without the grit and determination to continue. Whether or not we realised it at the time, by simply surviving the course, the characters remaining were self-selected prospective surgeons. It remained to be seen if the College examiners felt the same way.

At our final session with Stansfield, he finished the evening with a stirring crescendo. 'Gentlemen, I do not wish you luck because you won't need it. Instead, I wish you JUSTICE.'

The Royal College of Surgeons is a large impressive Georgian-styled building, all columns and tall windows, standing on the south side of Lincoln's Inn Fields, London. It's open to the public who usually go there to visit the wonderful Hunterian Museum. If you turn left immediately upon entering the main entrance hall, you will find a majestic white marble staircase descending to the cloakrooms and toilets in the basement. The area at the bottom of the stairs is large enough to hold twenty adults comfortably, or fifty at a crush, if they spill partway up the steps. The building and examination process – examiners versus examinees, numbers of prepared corpses and dissections – can accommodate around fifty candidates a day. With hundreds of applicants, the whole examination would last a week.

The College always notifies the candidates of their result with a simple "pass" or "fail" by post, but traditionally a list of the successful ones would be read out by the doorman or porter on the evening of each examination day. This was done from the top of the marble staircase. How the practice came about, or why it should be the responsibility of the College doorman, of all people, to deliver the bad news, I don't know. Nevertheless, after several hours hanging around Lincolns Inn Fields on a warm sunny afternoon, at the appointed time I joined the silent crush of fifty hopefuls in the cloakroom, and the doorman, in a smart Edwardian frock coat with silver buttons, duly appeared at the top of the stairs. He didn't shout names because we were all anonymous numbers, and the bad news came in the gaps, 'One zero five; one one one; one one three; one one nine ...' The crowd dwindled rapidly as the "gaps" filtered back up the stairs towards the exit, taking their lead from second or third-time failures who knew the drill. Those whose number was read out held back with the rest, unsure of what to do next. Around me were a handful of chums from the course, and we weren't going anywhere. As our individual numbers came up, we punched each other playfully in the ribs and whispered, 'Well done.' When the doorman disappeared without further instruction, we meandered to the local pub, intent on drunken debauchery, but the failures had arrived there before us. It didn't seem right to be celebrating at the same bar where they were drowning their sorrows, so instead we made our goodbyes, left for our respective homes, and got drunk there instead.

In the sober light of morning, it was a job well done. Passing the Primary at first attempt put me on the ladder to a surgical career, but it came at a price. Postgraduate exams and intensive training courses cost a small fortune, and the anatomy demonstrator job paid less than proper full-time doctoring. Even that was about to finish. Pre-clinical undergraduates have long summer holidays, so I wasn't required to teach anatomy and certainly didn't wish to learn any more. What me and my bank account desperately needed was to get back to clinical work and earn some decent money as a junior surgeon.

By then, it was early summer and jobs began on the 1st of August. That's every type of job, everywhere in the Britain, starting on the first day of August or February and lasting for six months or a multiple thereof. Imagine it: thousands of junior doctors playing a massive game of musical chairs twice a year, finishing at five or later in Cornwall and starting at nine or earlier in Cumbria, the next day. It was chaos on a huge scale with an inevitable amount of carnage thrown in. The message for the unwary was to avoid being a patient during the first week of the changeover. Not much has altered, though I understand the day is now fixed as the first Wednesday of the month rather than the first day.

With about six weeks to find something, I scoured the ads in the back pages of the British Medical Journal. It was a choice between SHO (senior house officer) in a teaching hospital where I'd be totally supervised/suffocated by juniors higher up the ladder wanting to do all the operating, or junior registrar in a district general hospital where I'd be less supervised, do a lot of operating, but risk being forgotten by the teaching hospital hierarchy. The safe option was SHO, spoon-fed with no opportunity to make my own decisions and learn. The brave option was junior registrar. But was I good enough not to screw up?

The dilemma was resolved with a phone call. I was in the Anatomy Department office reading a newspaper instead of a textbook. Pete was about two years ahead of me, went to the same medical school, played in the same soccer team as a rugged midfielder to my scrawny left-wing, had done the same anatomy demonstrator job, and had faced the same conundrum. He began with congratulations.

'How do you know? It was only last week.'

'Good news travels fast. Now, listen to me. You'll be wanting a job and there's one coming up here.'

'Yeah, I saw it in the BMJ, but that's a junior reg', Pete, and I'm not sure I'm up to it.'

'Don't be bloody stupid, you're perfect. Just what we need.'

'Who's we?'

'Me and the other registrars. Do you remember Joe Armitage?'

'What, Joe the goalie?'

'The very same. It's his post being advertised. He's just passed FRCS and got a reg' job at the Royal Free. He remembers you too and thinks you're just the man. You won't know the other guy because he's from Cardiff, but he's a good bloke. Come and see us, it's not that far.'

A few days later and an hour's drive to the suburbs of Sussex, we met in The Greyhound, a rural pub within walking distance of the hospital. The gorgeous summer evening tempted us into the beer garden where we could talk in relative peace and quiet. David Sleap (the Welshman) was with Pete; Joe was operating in theatre, but would join us if he could get away. They bombarded me with ale and information. Three firms, three registrars, three housemen, a one-in-three rota. All the juniors lived on the hospital site, either in flats (a small rent to the hospital) or a room (free in the residency block), so if you ran into trouble in theatres, your fellow registrars would be instantly available to help.

'But I've only done a handful of appendixes and hernias, and most of them were with a consultant or registrar.'

They glanced at each other and guffawed. I felt like an outsider being allowed an insight into a secret society. 'That's the whole point, boyo,' Dave explained in his soft musical accent. 'We've all done bugger all when we get here. The bosses know that and so do we. One of us ...' wagging a finger between himself and Pete, 'will always be around when you're on call. After a couple of months, you'll have learnt and done all the emergency stuff. And once a week you get to do your own list alongside the boss. Hernias, veins, odds and sods. It's bloody brilliant, man!'

Pete leaned forward to fix me with a serious frown. 'Look, emergencies are simple. When you boil it down, there are only five things you need to be able to do.' He counted them off on his fingers, 'Appendix, raise a colostomy, put a tube into a hot gall bladder, oversew a perf duodenal ulcer, and resect small bowel. Once you've learnt them, you can pretty much cope with anything. And what's more …' he paused for effect and grinned, 'if, when you're not on call, instead of bunking off to screw your latest girlfriend, you hang around and come to theatre with us instead, you'll get to do that lot in a couple of weeks, not months.'

The landlord came over with three more pints and plonked them down, spilling beer through the lattice of the wooden table onto the grass below. Overhead, chattering swallows carved aerobatics through the sultry evening air, heavy with the scent of flowerbeds and freshly mown grass. This quick trip to the sticks was turning out to be surprisingly pleasant. 'There you go lads, have these on me.' My two hosts exchanged pleasantries with Haitch (for Harold), an ageing wide-boy, heart-of-gold, cockney gentleman. He wore a West Ham football shirt to attract trade and hide his belly, rather than display any true allegiance to the club. His first love was always golf. Decades later, I would amputate one of his legs for diabetic gangrene. He died from a heart attack a few years afterwards and I attended the funeral.

'Is this the latest recruit, Peter?' Haitch tipped his head in my direction.

'Not quite, Haitch, but we're working on it.'

He winked at us and smiled. 'You know what lads, I've been watching this 'ere beer-in-the-garden interview for more years than I can remember, and I ain't never not seen the new bloke again. I reckon it's a done deal.' Haitch winked again, this time at me, 'See you soon,' and took the empty glasses back to the bar.

By the end of the evening, most of my cowardly reservations had been quashed and I'd been persuaded to, 'At least apply for the job.'

A couple of weeks later, I faced a more formal interview with the senior consultant surgeon in his office. Bill Packard asked the usual banal questions, and I gave the standard replies. When asked how much cutting I'd done, I was honest. He said that was how he liked it – I wasn't yet spoiled. Protocol required I wear a suit and tie rather than casual clothes, but I later discovered it wouldn't have mattered if I'd been stark naked. The deal had indeed been done. I'd been sucked into a surgeon factory, the most junior recruit always found and recommended to the chief by the incumbent registrars. He occasionally swallowed hard, particularly if it was a woman, but never rejected the registrars' choice. After all, at least one of them knew the applicant well (in my case, Pete) and was prepared to work with, and teach him, otherwise it might reflect badly on that registrar and the other. It was a system that had worked well for twenty years, except when his young protégés couldn't attract anyone with the right stuff. Rugby players were best, but a footballer or cricketer would do, a connection to his own alma mater – St Mary's – was regarded well, but above all, they needed to have passed the Primary at first attempt. Not much to ask perhaps, but on the few occasions when forced to make his own choice, 'I picked a few bummers,' as ex-RAF consultant surgeons are inclined to say.

I absorbed all this information over the following two

years in the post. In retrospect, Bill Packard preferred team players simply because it worked. Surgery is much like a team sport with a captain – the chief – and his players, all bonding by getting their kit off to change into team colours in the theatre changing room, and then repeating it in reverse after the game. Instead of numbered shirts and studded boots, it's theatre greens and clogs or white wellies, but without the stale sweat, mud and sharp smell of liniment oil. Other than that, there's little difference between a surgical changing room and a sporting one; they're both tips, strewn with clothes, footwear, dirty kit and towels. There's no doubt such intimacy promotes loyalty and team spirit, and it's a great leveller to be having a serious chat with the boss while he's wearing nothing but his old stringy piss-stained Y-fronts.

These days, the consultant does most of the one-to-one training, usually on juniors he barely knows, because the European Working Time Directive has been the death of team working and seriously marred surgical training. Back then, it was an era of so-called "see one, do one, teach one" surgery, when a barely competent junior surgeon was free to pass on his limited experience to another, and so on. With a trio of like-minded registrars on Packard's training conveyor belt, if he taught an operation to one of them, the wily old fox knew his efforts would be redoubled elsewhere, usually in the middle of the night or at weekends. With the other two consultants doing the same thing, the learning curve for the most junior team member was exponential.

Within a few months, as promised and delivered by Pete

and Welsh Dave, being on call was transformed from a fearful trek into the unknown to a joyous adventure of discovery. My two ever-present wingmen gently pulled back until I was flying on my own. Of the five need-to-know emergency procedures, appendicectomy was a once or twice daily event; the septic hot gall bladder, perf DU, and colostomy, once a fortnight; and resection of dead small bowel around once a month. There was lots of other minor stuff as well: abscesses, prolapsed piles, twisted testicles, and patients who needed surgical care rather than surgery. It was a busy job and I thrived with each new challenge. Some things clearly needed the boss to attend or make a decision: leaking aneurysms, chest trauma, post-operative bleeding, recurrent malignant obstruction, to name a few. I was happy to call him because we both knew they were beyond my experience and he was happy not to be bothered by trivia. In addition, I assisted and learned even more when he came in to do the big stuff, so it was win-win all round.

When I wasn't operating, I was reading surgical textbooks.

The Acute Abdomen for the Man on the Spot (first print 1965) was a little gem of a book written by a consultant surgeon sporting the incongruous name of Angell. Somewhat subversive in content, it was read widely by consultants and junior surgeons for at least two decades. The premise of the book was that during Angell's years of training, whenever he called one of his chiefs for help or advice regarding a patient, the request was met with something like, "You're the man on the spot old chap, I'm sure you're in the best position to do the right thing." Angell then went on, with macabre humour, to outline a series of acute abdomen scenarios with tips and hints for trainee surgeons on what to do and how to avoid or get out of difficulties.

I should explain an "acute abdomen" is surgical-speak for a patient presenting with severe abdominal pain, usually peritonitis (inflammation of the abdominal cavity), the cause of which is not immediately obvious from the history or clinical examination. Back in Angell's day, and at least half of mine, diagnostic scans didn't exist. It was plain X-ray, blood tests, an operation (look-see) or observation (wait-see), all underpinned by whatever degree of clinical acumen was available. Modern scanning techniques will visualise the abdomen and uncover its hidden secrets at the touch of a button, so the undiagnosed acute abdomen is long gone. But to give you an idea of what it was like in those not-so-far-off times, I'll share some of his advice regarding laparotomy, a look-see abdominal operation. It's paraphrased from memory and the parentheses are mine.

"You will at some stage be doing a laparotomy for an acute abdomen and yet after an exhaustive examination of every organ and every segment of bowel, will find nothing amiss. It might then occur to you that myocardial infarction [heart attack] *could well be the cause of the original abdominal pain. DO NOT share this thought with the anaesthetist; it will be met with a frenzy of panicked activity at the top end of the table*

and much abuse hurled in your direction. Rather, simply close the incision and quietly arrange for an electrocardiogram [ECG] *once the patient is in the recovery room."* You can see why it was popular.

A much heavier and learned tome was *Emergency Surgery* (first print 1930 – that's not a typo, it really was 1930) by Henry Hamilton Bailey, though the "Henry" was dropped from his publications. Hundreds of pages and many years of hands-on surgical know-how beautifully distilled into specific advice with illustrated instructions, *Hamilton Bailey's Emergency Surgery* has been used as a pillow by generations of trainee surgeons, sleeplessly waiting in the on-call bedroom for the phone or bleeper to announce the arrival of yet another challenge to their uncertain ability.

A&E doctor: 'I've got an old girl of eighty down here with a strangulated femoral hernia.'

Surgical Registrar, trying to sound competent: 'Okay, I'll be there in five.' Then, diving into his well-thumbed copy and muttering, 'Shit, shit, shit,' he'd find the appropriate section, complete with instructions, anatomic drawings and monochrome photos, and remind himself, possibly for the first time, how to do the operation.

Bailey died in 1961, but there isn't a British or English-speaking surgeon since 1930 who hasn't read his book. *Emergency Surgery* is still in print, edited by successive generations of surgical doyens with numerous contributors, each no doubt with personal memories of how Henry Hamilton Bailey helped them cope in the middle of many dark nights. Coincidently, the publisher's blurb for the 13th edition (2015) recommends the book as, "A definitive source for the surgeon on the spot". Clearly, at least one of the two editors had Angell's 1965 *Man on the Spot* book in mind.

Bailey wrote several other books, but one was produced in collaboration with another surgeon, a colleague called McNeil Love (died 1974). *Bailey and Love's Short Practice of Surgery* (first print 1932 – again, not a typo), about the size of a breeze block and anything but short, covered every imaginable surgical topic using logical readable text, memorable footnotes, amusing anecdotes, and like *Emergency Surgery* was littered with photos and illustrations. It's now in its 26th edition (2013).

Arguably, these two books have educated more surgeons than any other, past or present. To re-edit, update and publish the titles on a regular basis is a mammoth task for all concerned. For that I say thank you, and so will ranks of future surgeons.

The euphoric confidence in my ability to handle emergency surgery didn't last long.

Saturday afternoon and a twenty-year-old girl with what appeared to be appendicitis on the table. No problem. Easy peasy. Yet, the small right lower abdominal incision – small and low as possible for a girl – produced a torrent of blood. It was a Jesus moment, as in, 'Jesus, what the hell is this?' Cold sweat instantly trickled down my back, and beneath the face mask my cheeks flushed red hot. What to do? The anaesthetist, a short Asian guy and a junior like me, panicked too. We'd worked together often and I assumed he was a rock-steady bloke, but now, in a high-pitched voice, he was demanding cross-matched blood from the orderly while adding an inch or two to the skid marks in his pants. The commotion from the north end of the table had me feverishly extend the incision for a better view. Hamilton Bailey was guiding my thoughts: *If you can't do it through the hole you have, make a bigger hole.* Still no bleeding point, no hissing, pissing blood vessel. I hooked the appendix out for a look. *Normal, so leave it alone. Don't turn a clean operation into a potentially infected one.* Grabbing the sucker from my houseman, I placed it carefully into the depths of the pelvis and growled, 'Suck.'

A month previously, this might have been a Pete or Dave moment, but I recognised it was probably beyond their understanding as well as mine. Racking my brains for causes of a belly full of blood in a twenty-year-old girl without trauma, the only thing that went Ding! was hepatic adenoma, a rare and particularly vascular liver tumour with a nasty habit of spontaneously bleeding. This was a boss job, no question about it. But if I rang him now, I knew he'd tell me to do a proper laparotomy, yet the girl could be bleeding to death even while I was on the phone. The logical imperative was to find the source of bleeding and stop it, or at least press on it. Then, I could call for help. The scrub nurse was an experienced senior sister with about twenty years on me.

'Betty, I think we need a better look.'

The knife was ready in her hand. 'I'm sure that's what Mr N would do.'

Ignoring the appendicectomy hole, *it can always be used as a drain exit*, with a trembling hand I made a decent length up-and-down incision, examined everything in fine detail, particularly the liver, washed the blood from the abdomen with saline, and found ... absolutely nothing. So, I did it again with even greater care. Zilch. Time to call the boss.

'Check out her ovaries more carefully,' he said, after his wife dragged him from the lawn mower to the phone. 'You'll find a small bloody spot where she's recently ovulated and bled more excessively than normal. Give the ovary a squeeze and a squirt of blood should appear. It's probably not necessary now, but put in a good deep stitch to stop any more bleeding and Bob's your Uncle. Oh, and since she's going to be left with an appendix scar, at her age take out the appendix, it could save a helluva lot of confusion in the future.'

After scrubbing and gowning again, I went back into her abdomen. There it was, on the walnut-sized right ovary, exactly as he described. Gentle pressure produced a small blood clot followed by a thin fountain of scarlet. A simple stitch secured it. Ten minutes later, the appendix was out, and I began closing the abdomen, doing my best to be neat so the eventual scar wouldn't be too ugly. Either way the two scars amounted to a tick sign, *my* tick sign, and she would be wearing it for life, all for the sake of a tiny stitch in her ovary that took less than half a minute to do. I regarded the superficial result of my work of the previous hour and felt distraught. The boss knew what was going on down to the finest detail, over the phone, without even being there. How come I was so stupid? Why didn't I know?

Ovulation being associated with trivial minor bleeding is an accepted fact. Blood is an irritant in the abdominal cavity and many women experience mild mid-cycle discomfort when the developing follicle (Latin: *folliculus*; little bag) ruptures to release the egg. Vaginal spotting can also occur, presumably because blood in the pelvis exits via the fallopian tubes. For some women, the discomfort and spotting are sure and reliable signs of ovulation. But bleeding enough to flood the abdomen?

'It's rare, but it happens,' the boss said, when I tackled him a few days later on the ward round. The girl was recovering well. 'Have you checked her clotting and all the other stuff?' The clotting, including lots of other "stuff", were normal. When we were out of earshot, I pushed it further. 'Rare or not, you knew what it was.'

'Only because you excluded everything else, and I've seen it before.' His smile and tone invited further questioning.

'How often?'

'Just the once, and before you ask, yes, I did a laparotomy too.'

At this point, we shall have a short intermission in the account of my surgical training, because the following tale fits well with the one above and I can't think of a more appropriate place to put it. So, here we go ...

Many years later, whenever I was the on-call consultant, I developed a habit of checking theatres at the end of the day for anything that might need my attention. All too often, I'd left for home at seven, only to be called back just as I sat down to an evening meal. On one occasion, I found the duty registrar about to remove an appendix from a thirteen-year-old girl. Because the registrar was new and I'd not seen her operate before, I thought it prudent to change into greens and at least keep an eye on her. Besides, one can learn a lot from observing a junior surgeon in action, chiefly whether they're any good or not. Most are rubbish because they haven't yet done enough cutting to be confident, slick and quick. Rarely, perhaps two or three times in a career, one comes along with hands so full of magic it takes your breath away, like discovering an untutored child who's a genius at art or music. Never tell them though; it would spoil them. Simply supply more difficult work to develop confidence and boldness, and ever watchful, make sure they're not so overstretched it breaks their spirit.

Removing a hot appendix can be damn difficult at times, and if the registrar needed help it would save me a return trip. However, trying to operate with the boss breathing down your neck is very off-putting, so I sat down next to the anaesthetist, an old man like me, rested my weary knees and made small talk at the top end of the table while she cracked on at the business end. Within five minutes, the sucker was working overtime. 'Her abdomen is full of blood.'

My fellow geriatric dropped his shoulders and sighed to me, 'Whatever it is, she's not bleeding. This kid's stable as a brick. She's not even febrile.'

After giving the order to keep sucking, I scrubbed up and swapped places with the registrar. She walked around to the other side of the table, in turn displacing the houseman, another young woman, to the space on her right. The scrub nurse was Audrey, a senior sister who regularly did my aneurysms. Because her shift was due to finish at eight, she had one eye on the clock and the other on me, a result of complicated childcare arrangements. Unless there is a pressing need, having to swap a scrub nurse mid-operation is generally frowned upon because it's a recipe for confused swab and instrument counts. 'Don't worry Auds, I'll have you out of here well before eight – with plenty of time to put the kids to bed and let your mum get home.' Above the mask, her eyes gave me a thank you.

Of course, all the while, I had this operation sussed. Done it before hadn't I? "Just the once." But this time there'd be no laparotomy, no everlasting tick-shaped scar. That was until I took out the sucker and looked at the "blood". It was neither bright red (arterial) nor dark mauve (venous), but an odd pink-brown colour. I put two fingers deep into the wound and slurped out a good amount to wipe onto a clean white swab, then stared at it, not quite believing my eyes. The three women surrounding me agreed: it was menstrual blood. They hadn't recognised it in the clear plastic sucker tubing, but mingled with the cotton swab it was obvious. I looked to my left and saw two mounds beneath the green drapes, below me and to the right, pubic hair poked out from the lower sheet. This schoolgirl had boobs and pubes. 'When was her last period?' I asked the registrar. But she couldn't give me an answer.

'She's hasn't started yet,' the little houseman intervened, averting her gaze from mine for fear of upstaging the registrar.

I hooked out the appendix followed by the right ovary; both normal. Reaching across to the left side, blindly searching with the tips of two fingers for the other ovary, I bumped into a twelve-week sized uterus, as big as a large avocado. *It can't be – she can't be pregnant, surely not?* 'Is she sexually active? Pregnancy test result?' The registrar stared blankly at me again. Bloody useless, she should have known.

'Urine test negative. I didn't bother to ask about boyfriends,' the houseman answered once more, but 'boyfriends' was spat out like a posh gob of phlegm aimed at me, or possibly all men in general.

Beneath my mask, I couldn't help but smile to myself. She was good and knew it, but I couldn't let it pass. Her tone meant she assumed a girl of thirteen wouldn't have a sexual partner so didn't enquire, and that it was outrageously vulgar and utterly distasteful for any man, particularly one of my age, to even consider the possibility. The urine pregnancy test was part of the routine screening done by the A&E nurses, so the aggrieved Miss Prim houseman could lay no claim to it, other than she knew the result and the registrar didn't.

In despair at the naïve ignorance, I gave out a great sigh followed by a few huffs and puffs, just for emphasis. 'Last week on the TOP (Termination of Pregnancy) list was a mother and her twelve-year-old daughter, both impregnated by Mum's boyfriend. And last year, there was another double act, but in that case the daughter's boyfriend was the culprit. He was fifteen, she was fourteen and her mother was thirty-five.' This was entirely true. I upped the volume a little for effect, 'All females with boobs and pubes are pregnant until proved otherwise. Got it?' The little houseman nodded vigorously in the glow of my benign malevolence. The registrar knew she was in for a bollocking. But that would come later, and in private.

The hiatus of scolding the juniors, though lasting less than half a minute, was purposeful; it taught them a lesson and gave me time to think. The experienced consultant anaesthetist had already assured me the girl wasn't actively bleeding and was stable. On impulse, I dragged out the right ovary again, along with the top end of the fallopian tube, and with the other hand pressed on the unusually enlarged, but unexplained, uterus. Pink-brown menstrual blood poured through the tube into my gloved palm. This child was menstruating backwards into her abdomen. Given her age and post-pubescent state, she must have been in regular agony for a year or more.

'Audrey,' I said to the scrub nurse, 'You're gonna hate me for this, but we need to check out her undercarriage, and it won't be sterile. Let's pull her knees up with her ankles together for a good look.' It was a bit of a kerfuffle, but with a few additional green drapes we kept the appendix wound sterile, adjusted the overhead light and inspected her perineum.

Protruding from her vagina and nestling between the labia was a small mauve balloon, the size of the pulp of my thumb. I'd guessed correctly, it was an imperforate hymen. A normal virginal hymen has an aperture through which menses and trivial amounts of mucus flow out. This kid must have been blocked up since birth. 'Poor girl,' Audrey whispered to herself, but the two juniors were dumbstruck. I suppose only women could truly appreciate the child's predicament. In my line of work, I'd never seen one. It was uncommon, but nevertheless, something needed to be done. I briefly considered the politically correct option of calling for a gynaecologist, and then spent even less time dismissing the thought. We would have been there for hours and my previous experiences with the specialty generally filled me with awe of the wrong kind. There was also Audrey's mum and her children's bedtime to consider. 'Let's have a white needle and syringe, Auds.'

Using the largest (colour-coded white) hypodermic needle, I pierced the dome of the "balloon" at its most prominent point and drew back the plunger. The syringe filled with the same coloured fluid that was sloshing around the abdomen. Good, now I had somewhere safe to cut: nothing but menstrual blood lay just beyond that specific part of the paper-thin hymen. I enlarged the pinprick a couple of millimetres with a blade and tore through the rest with an implement that couldn't possibly do any harm, the tip of my little finger. Audrey recognised the plan and pushed a kidney dish between the girl's buttocks. 'Ready?' She nodded and caught the gush of fluid as my finger withdrew. In all, it amounted to about half a pint.

After scrubbing again, I checked the uterus had deflated to normal size, removed the appendix to save a "helluva lot of confusion in the future", washed out the abdomen with saline and sewed her up. In all, it was a good evening's work. Audrey made it to her kids on time, I had my dinner at a reasonable hour, and the new registrar received some constructive, but memorably loud advice. 'It's morally, ethically, and probably criminally negligent to operate on a patient unless you know all the pertinent facts about the case. That includes the test results, the sexual history, and if needs be, their grandmother's maiden name and her fucking inside leg measurement. Don't EVER do it again.'

The child recovered from surgery exceptionally well, with only a small appendix scar to show for it. Before handing her over to the gynaecologists, I told the houseman to have a girly chat with the patient regarding her newfound womanhood and how to deal with it.

Two years after the girl with the bleeding ovary frightened the life out of me on a Saturday afternoon, I'd done eighteen months of general surgery and six months of orthopaedics. General surgery introduced me to the sub-specialities of urology, vascular, upper gastro-intestinal (oesophagus and stomach), lower GI (colon and rectum), and breast and endocrine (mostly thyroids). Orthopaedic carpentry introduced me to boredom and a world of intellectual destitution. In addition to elective surgery sessions and out-patient clinics, I was on a one-in-three on-call rota dealing with all general surgery and orthopaedic emergencies. That's 243 days and nights, or 5,832 hours.

Elective surgery lists were organised by the registrars. Each Monday, I'd take a trip to the admissions office to pick patients off the waiting list for operating sessions the following week. The waiting list itself was a small grey filing cabinet with long, thin pull-out drawers, each containing a dozen or more admission slips showing the patients' details and the operation that needed scheduling. These ranged from "urgent" in the top drawers (usually cancers or children), down through "soon" (duodenal ulcer or gallstone ops for example), to the most humdrum "routine" (lumps and bumps, hernias, varicose veins) in the lowest drawers. The urgent cases reflected the special interest of whichever boss I was working for at the time (mastectomy, aneurysm, prostatectomy, colon resection) but the "soon" and "routine" were standard general surgery fodder. For a junior registrar with his own operating list to fill, it was like being a kid in a sweet shop. In the early days, I foraged in the lowest drawers where I could probably do no harm – fatty lumps, skin cysts, small hernias and the like. As time went by, I slowly worked my way up the filing cabinet until, towards the end of my tenure, I was comfortable with most things.

On one occasion, I took it too far. With nothing urgent on the waiting list that week, I scheduled a list full of varicose veins for the boss. Meanwhile, in the adjoining theatre I'd put together a decent registrar list for my own amusement –

a gallbladder, duodenal ulcer and a couple of hernias.

Before the morning's work began, the boss stormed in to see me. 'Tell me, all those varicose veins on my list, are they private?' He was not amused.

'Er, what do you mean?' I was bewildered.

'Are they private patients?'

'No, at least … not as far as I know. They're off your waiting list.' *Meaning: they're your patients, how am I supposed to know if they're private or not?*

'Well, that's a great pity. You see, I only do private varicose veins because I'm allergic to any other sort. So, you're going next door to do them, while I stay here and do your list.'

It was an important lesson. Never again give the chief mind-numbing varicose vein surgery. Boring stuff is the sole preserve of the registrar.

As the months passed into years, first Pete and then Welsh Dave passed FRCS at first try and moved on to proper registrar posts in London teaching hospitals. I'd helped to pick both their successors in The Greyhound beer garden interview, done my bit to shepherd them through the first few months of on-call and slowly became the senior man in our little dynasty. Somehow and somewhere along the way, I managed to become a half-decent clinician and surgeon.

I'll never forget a couple of insights Dave imparted to me late one evening in the doctors' mess bar. Pete was on call, so we were free to have a few beers and enjoy our night off. The first involved his preference for skinny girlfriends.

'It must be like going to bed with a cattle grid, Dave. Why do you like them so slim?'

'Because, boyo, the meat is sweetest nearest the bone.'

It was both a prophetic statement and a Freudian slip. His true passion was bones and he went on to become an orthopaedic consultant. The second insight, inevitably, was about surgery.

'The trick is, see, any pillock can surge himself into trouble, but bloody good surgeons can surge themselves out of it. That's the difference.'

After two years and all that on-call time, I'd reached the point, at least in those operations within my scope, where I could "surge" myself out of trouble. Of course, the real trick is not to arrive there in the first place; that takes anticipation and experience. I was nowhere near that nirvana but was ready to attempt the next rung on the ladder, final FRCS. Like the Primary, it involved expensive examination fees and another course.

Whipps Cross Hospital, or simply Whipps, as it's known in the trade, lies in the north-east suburbs of London and has run final FRCS courses for as long as anyone can remember. Back then, it was a rather sprawling semi-rural district general hospital within spacious manicured grounds, but with strong historic ties to London teaching hospitals. Consequently, although the course was hosted by the Whipps' surgeons, they were also joined by superstars from the big city, most of whom were famous professors or college examiners. It was *the* course to get on but required sponsorship – a recommendation of suitability – from your present boss. The pass rate was astronomically high and, presumably, the organisers didn't want their statistics ruined by people attempting the exam too soon. In the event, around fifty were accepted and many were also Slome-Stansfield graduates.

The two-week course was an intensive revision of all we were expected to know. Various luminaries led us through the minutiae of what amounted to their individual hobby, while better teachers simplified the complex. Clinical sessions with volunteer patients showed us how to impress with the routine, and startle with the rarities. It ran with the ruthless testosterone-fuelled efficiency of an army boot camp. Being told by an eminent professor, "You're as useless as a perforated condom," must be good for a surgeon's soul – though it wasn't just me; most of us gained similar accolades. To give a flavour of the intensity, I need only to tell you about the course leader: a neat slim man who demanded neat slim responses to his questions. I understand he once took a phone call from his wife in the middle of a ward round. All the juniors waited attentively around the nurses' desk as he conversed on the landline. The following is a rough transcription of half the verbal exchange as overheard and relayed to me:

'What do you mean, a leak? Is it gas or water?'

'Hot or cold?'

'How much?'

'"Lots," doesn't tell me much. Is it a slow drip, a gallon a minute, a creeping flood, a raging torrent?'

'Where's it coming from?'

'Yes, it would be on the floor, but which room? Which floor?'

'Right. Have you checked the ceiling, under the sink, toilet, shower, radiator?'

'Mmm ... call an emergency plumber.'

'Yellow Pages.'

In fairness, the Whipps' course was spectacularly good, the content and delivery perfect for guys at our stage (again, I recall no women). Viva practice was a far worse interrogation than the wife with plumbing problems received, and as I've demonstrated above, the pithy put-downs were unforgettable.

Either way, the formula worked, because a few weeks later several perforated condoms found themselves once more in the crush outside the toilets at the foot of the Royal College staircase. This time, the porter read out the numbers but made sure the successful candidates stayed behind after the failures trudged up the stairs to the exit. We were then led to a large hall where all the examiners were lined up in splendid scarlet gowns worn over their suits. One by one, we shuffled down the line, shook hands, were given a repeated, 'Well done,' and then directed to a secretary at a desk who demanded a cheque for £200 to cover the cost of annual College membership. It was bad timing at best and planned robbery in the extreme, particularly coming on top of the expense of the exam and the course. After all, who among us was going to object? Who could even afford it? My elation at passing evaporated in an indignant fury. Surely such a bill should come in the post, along with the certificate. I wasn't alone. Those of us who'd already signed and passed over our cheque gathered at one end of the hall and were soon joined by the rest, perhaps a dozen in all. The examiners crowded at the other end, still in their finery, and outnumbered us. Our whispered general feeling was: screw'em, we've done it, we're FRC bloody ESSES, so let's get out of here and get drunk. We may have been offered sherry and small talk, but quite truthfully, I remember nothing else of that evening.

The following morning, I awoke in the bed of my hospital flat, safely in one piece but suffering a hangover from hell, with yesterday's smart suit and tie a crumpled mess on the bedroom floor. Nevertheless, by seven-thirty I was triple-essed (shit, showered, shaved), wearing fresh clothes, a clean white coat, and sitting in the almost-deserted hospital canteen, drowning myself in heavily sugared black coffee. The houseman joined me at the table where we always met to plan the day. Tony was a delightfully amusing free spirit, and an equally liberal Jew. He passed me a greasy bacon sandwich with the instruction, 'Eat it. It'll either kill or cure,' and began tucking into his own. We'd discussed his penchant for bacon before, 'I like it and the scriptures are out of date, so I won't get tapeworms.' I guessed his public boarding school education lifted him above the rigid confines of any religion.

'You don't remember much of last night, do you?' It was a statement of fact.

'No,' I admitted.

'Mess bar, midnight, drinks on you?'

'Sounds plausible, Tony, but fuck knows how I got there.'

'A taxi dumped you outside the mess. You must have taken the train from town and a cab from the station.'

'How pissed was I?'

'Not too bad. When you arrived, I'd say halfway between happily merry and shitfaced. But then we dragged you into the bar, poured champagne down your neck, and the rest, as they say, is history.'

'Bastards.'

'Then, we put you to bed.'

'Thanks.'

So that was it. I was a bona fide surgeon. Once the girls on the switchboard knew, they called me "Mister" rather than "Doctor" and the rest of the hospital followed suit. The peculiarly British tradition of surgeons being addressed as Mister confuses many patients: "I wanna see a proper Doctor, norra Mister," is a frequent cry.

It originated centuries ago when qualified physicians holding university doctorates delegated such brutality to the local barber, who was called upon to lance boils, pull teeth and other, more adventurous interventions, such as amputation. Seen in every town and street today, the striped red and white pole outside a barbershop still signifies blood and bandages, rather than a place to get a haircut. To cut a long story short, the barber-surgeons organised themselves, got their act into gear and were eventually awarded a Royal Charter, but kept the title Mister because they didn't hold a doctorate. There's still a London City Livery Company of Barber-Surgeons, and what's more, the Royal College of Surgeons is an offshoot of the Barber-Surgeons' guild. I'd gone from Mr Student to Dr Inexperienced to Mr Surgeon in the space of four years.

But I knew it was only the beginning. In effect, I'd passed the driving test for surgery and held a licence, so could throw the L-plates away. Competence at an operating table would need many more years of practice and training.

There is an ironic twist to this tale. About twenty years after the RCS awarded me the Fellowship with one hand and callously robbed me blind with the other, leaving me so angry and resentful it ruined what should have been a gloriously triumphant day, they asked me to become an examiner. By nature, I'm wary of such establishments – GMC and BMA included – for much the same reason I'm wary of career politicians who've never held down a proper job. My impression is that they tend to attract vain, pompous, self-seeking individuals with political ambitions, rather than those with a fervent calling to selfless public service. True, council members are democratically elected by their peers, but for many I think it's their ego and ambition which pushes them to stand. In equal measure, deep down, the ire I felt on the day of my own examination still niggled two decades after the event. As a result, the request to join the throng gave me mixed feelings, with a strong inclination to refuse the honour.

I took advice from an older colleague who'd already

served his time on the Court of Examiners. 'Best club you'll ever belong to. Bloody hard work, but the evening dinners and booze-ups are legendary. You'll meet a lot of friends you haven't seen in years and make loads of new ones. Plus – and it's a big plus – being a gatekeeper for excellence is an extremely rewarding task. I know your opinion of the College, but examiners have nothing much to do with those characters, and most of the chaps I met feel the same way as you. I think you're perfect for it. Why not give it a go? You can easily resign, but I know you'll enjoy it.'

As he spoke, I looked him straight in the eye and realisation dawned. 'You've put me up for this, haven't you?'

'Yes,' he giggled.

I served for about eight years, including wearing the scarlet robes at the end of each long and exhausting day. It was all he said it would be, and more. My reward was the deep satisfaction of knowing only the absolutely best candidates were given a pass and would go on to even greater achievements. It truly was an honour to play my part. But then again, there were never any demands for annual membership fees to spoil the celebrations.

Now, I need to acknowledge the surgeon's unsung heroine, or increasingly common hero, the scrub nurse. I briefly mentioned Betty earlier, the scrub nurse with me on the Saturday I carved an indelible tick scar into a young woman's abdomen. I'm certain every surgeon in the world has their own special version of Betty. She'd been working in theatres for almost as long as I'd been alive when I started:

a wet behind the ears twenty-five-year-old of doubtful ability and zero experience, contrasted with a senior sister who'd scrubbed for more surgeons and more surgery than I'd ever see in a lifetime. Betty always worked the night shift or weekends because it fitted in with her husband's day job and childcare. Consequently, whenever I was operating on out-of-hours emergencies she was always there, either scrubbed for the big stuff or overseeing the work of one of her own junior nurses when it was something simple like an abscess or appendix.

During my two pre-FRCS learning years, I like to think she saw some ability in me to which I was perpetually blind, or perhaps she'd dealt with so many similar imbeciles she could manage the incompetence. Either way, Betty taught, encouraged, emboldened, and sometimes harangued me into doing the right operation or making the correct decision, most often at three in the morning. 'Mr P would use this ...' passing me a particular instrument or clamp, or, 'No, Mr N doesn't like that – he prefers this suture.' I soon learned to turn it around, 'Betty, what would Mr J do, use, prefer, say, cut next?' And she always knew. In truth, the surgical skills I attained were as much her doing as any of my medically qualified peers or chiefs. Sadly, not many years into retirement she developed cancer, and all too-quickly went the way of all flesh. So, here's to Betty with love, and all her wonderful kind.

6

A LAD WITH ULCERATIVE COLITIS

At home, in the poky spare bedroom that doubles as an office and unofficial storeroom for unwieldy household appliances – today, it's the vacuum cleaner, ironing board and an indoor contraption for airing clothes – I have on the wall a large framed certificate. It's there at the behest of the owner/operator of the appliances that clutter the floor. She found it in an old filing cabinet in the garage where it had lain undisturbed for decades, rolled inside a long cardboard tube. 'It'll look nice,' she pleaded, before interpreting my drooping head as consent. For anyone who cares to read it, in copperplate script together with a faux red wax seal, it declares that I have completed, "*... the training required both in surgery in general and in the specialty of GENERAL SURGERY to the satisfaction of ...*" Issued by the Royal College of Surgeons, London (the upper case and tautology are theirs), and signed by several notable surgeons, it is dated 1987, the year I started my consultant job as a *vascular* surgeon. How does that work? Let me explain.

Fifty years ago, or more, unless you were a specialist plastic, orthopod, neuro, eye, O&G, ENT, cardiothoracic, or maxillofacial surgeon (warning: this list is not exhaustive and may not be entirely accurate), by default you were a generalist with a special interest in whatever. The reason I can't be entirely accurate with the specialist list back then is simple: at one time, every surgeon was a generalist, trained in all of the above and free to tackle any of them, producing predictably diverse results. Those who were worse in one or more sphere of activity avoided them; those who were better, avoided the others. Thus, by a form of Darwinian natural selection, specialists grew like tall weeds in the low-lying pasture fields of generalists. Before long, the tall weeds attracted acolytes who, having been trained by the master, scattered like seeds among the pasture and grew tall themselves. Being both sociable and thirsty, like-minded weeds formed friendly societies to wine and dine, disseminate knowledge, promote education and training, and lobby the appropriate authority to recognise their expertise as "specialist".

Search "Father of Modern ... *name of specialty*," and you'll be rewarded with the life history of a recognised doyen. Cushing (of Cushing's Disease) for neurosurgery, Thomas (of the Thomas splint) for orthopaedics, Gillies (Gillies' forceps) or McIndoe (eponymous scissors inventor and patron of the Guinea Pig Club) for plastic surgery, to name but a few. I haven't done it, but I suspect if you perform the same search in a language other than English, you'll get different seminaries for differing countries.

But what stimulates the growth of a specialty, or a specialist? For millennia it has most often been war, forever a catalyst of human inventiveness. Hippocrates advised, "He who wishes to be a surgeon should go to war," and armies have forever employed some sort of surgeon to mop up the casualties. However, we'll stick with more recent conflicts.

Harvey Cushing, for example, an American general surgeon with a growing interest in neurology and neurosurgery, became embroiled in the European theatre of the First World War (1914–18). Before the adoption of steel helmets, penetrating skull (brain) injuries were lethal, but the helmets rendered them survivable. For the first time, soldiers arrived in field hospitals alive, but with bits of metal causing havoc within their brain: enter Cushing, who improved the surgical treatment and halved the death rates. Similarly, mortality from fractures of the femur fell from 80% to 20% due to the Thomas splint, which stabilised the injury. Burnt British and allied airmen had their faces and hands reconstructed (World War 2) by McIndoe because they were falling out of the sky onto home turf rather than enemy-occupied foreign territory. His innovative and experimental techniques helped many severely disfigured servicemen, who formed the famous Guinea Pig Club in his honour. Modern vascular surgery arguably has its origins in the Korean War (1950–53), when it became common practice amongst military surgeons to defy standing orders (presumably under threat of Court Martial) and repair damaged limb arteries rather than simply cut the arm or leg off. Post-war, all the experience and learning garnered from treating battle injuries of every kind was transferred to civilian practice, where it stimulated the growth of specialties, though it might be many years until the governing bodies recognised them as such. For example, my own consultant job was advertised as "General surgeon with a special interest in vascular surgery", but twenty-five years later, vascular surgery was finally granted individual specialty status.

The peacetime route to develop a special interest is to be a general surgeon doing fixed weekly sessions in a mixed out-patient department (OPD), something we all do as part of the job. An OPD can have a dozen or more consulting rooms, each occupied by a consultant in any specialty you care to name, but the trick is, they're all there at the same time each and every week, and they know you are too. Many superb thyroid surgeons developed the skill simply because each week they did a clinic next door to an endocrinologist (hormone physician). I spent twenty-five years doing clinics alongside experts in neurology, rheumatology, gastroenterology, dentistry, ENT, nephrology, gynaecology, oncology, haematology, dermatology, and a few more I've forgotten because they never bothered me, and I never bothered them. Consequently, I became the go-to man for skin, nerve and muscle biopsy, temporal artery biopsy, lymph gland biopsy, and other urgent diagnostic procedures. Along the way, I became adept at removing huge spleens for the haematologist, forming arterio-venous shunts (for haemodialysis) for the nephrologist, and excising inflammatory bowel disease for the gastroenterologist.

Wee Willie was one such patient.

It began, as these things do, with a tap on the door of my OPD room. Peter Newton, the short stout gastroenterologist from across the corridor, pushed it ajar and put his head through the gap, 'Have you got a couple of minutes?' I was between patients and he knew it; the nurse outside would have told him. 'Sure. What is it?' I said, getting up from behind my desk.

'Come and see,' he tipped his head to beckon me.

Newton led the way back to his own room. A little older than me, he'd been a consultant for five years or so, whereas I'd only just started. Despite a reputation for being grumpy and direct, he was an excellent clinician and shit-hot with an endoscope inserted in the top or bottom end. 'It's a lad with ulcerative colitis. I've only recently inherited him from the paediatricians but he's not doing well. Right now, he's having a bit of a relapse so I'm about to admit him for a few days' intensive treatment, but I think it's time for a colectomy. What I want to know is can we do it here, or do I need to send him into town?' *Meaning: "Are you capable of performing such an operation or will he need to go to a London teaching hospital?"*

The boy and his mum were sitting side by side in front of Newton's desk. Mum looked frazzled, the boy looked pale and pasty, with the typical puffed-out face of steroid treatment. Short, skinny and prepubertal, he appeared to be about eleven or twelve years old. I perched half my bum on the corner of the desk, introduced myself with a handshake, and then glanced at the thick wad of notes, primarily to ascertain his name.

'Now then, William, how old are you?'

'Please call me Will or Willie, only teachers call me William.' He spoke with the assurance of an older child. I reasoned it was because he'd been dealing with white coats like me for years, so didn't feel shy or intimidated.

I smiled. 'Sorry about that. Let's start again. Willie, how–'

'I'm sixteen, but look much younger.'

Jeez. My immediate thought was the poor little tyke must be bullied to death at school. For sixteen, he was a complete runt and his peers would be young men in comparison. Mum read my face and quietly nodded, recognising I understood and shared her concerns. Popping Will on the couch, I quickly checked him over: anaemic, dehydrated, underweight, belly soft, no scars, no pain, skin like warm thin dough – steroids again. The surgery itself wouldn't be a problem, his chronic ill health and lack of physical resilience would be. Plus the damn steroids, of course; poor healing, more infection, less resistance. Then I excused myself and Newton into the corridor for a private chat.

'Well?' Newton raised his eyebrows.

I was quietly seething. 'That kid should have been done ages ago. He needs a colectomy and to be off the steroids. Nothing fancy though. A simple colectomy and ileostomy. No pouch. He needs to grow before that's even a consideration. I think he'll be better off without a mucous fistula too, as long as you're happy to treat his rectal stump. If you need a fistula, he can have one, but I think the ileostomy will be more than enough for him to handle. I also think you'll have to manage his steroid withdrawal and fluid balance bloody carefully, and post-op he'll need ITU for a day or two to be on the safe side.'

'You'll do it then?' Newton grinned at my implicit assent.

'Pete, he's better off here with me and you, rather than a couple of half-wit senior registrars in town. But I do mean me, *and* you. If you abandon him, he'll fall through the cracks with an Addisonian crisis or worse. Post-op he could be a bloody nightmare. You know it.'

'I totally agree. And I'll be with him, *and* you, every step. The big question is, when?'

I'd already thought it through. 'Will next Wednesday's morning list give you enough time to get him up to speed?'

'That'll do nicely. Perfect. And thanks.'

'Good. You get him in, sort him out, and I'll chat up ITU and the anaesthetist. If he goes downhill before then, I'll do him on an emergency list.'

Before explaining ulcerative colitis (UC), I need to say a few things about our intimately close but often forgotten friend, the colon. Also known as the large intestine, it's the last four foot or so of bowel that terminates at the rectum and anus. Unlike the simple uniform tube of the much longer small intestine, the colon resembles a string of sausages with multiple bulges, or at least that's what we all thought when examining that anatomy poster at school. Whereas the small intestine digests and absorbs our foodstuff, the colon functions as a raw sewage processor. Waste material, undigested food and many litres of fluid enter at one end, conveniently solid faeces exit at the other, and in between most of the water is extracted. It all sounds beguilingly simple and our everyday experience reinforces this impression. But of course, it's not.

Firstly, because the internal lining of the colon has many visible folds and creases, and at a microscopic level there are multitudes of further folds and creases, the total internal surface area is huge, enabling it to efficiently absorb large volumes of water. It's an oddity in medicine that such exponential increases in surface area are usually described, for memorable effect, as equating to the size of a ball-game area. So as not to break with tradition, let's just say you could have a slimy game of tennis on your spread-out colon.

Secondly, the colon – with no exaggeration – is home to trillions of bacteria of several hundred varieties. These digest and ferment what we can't, notably plant fibre, and feed on it. More "fibre" in our diet makes us "regular" because it feeds the bacteria. The bran in your breakfast muesli or cereal nourishes the bugs and boosts their numbers, which in turn bulks up the size of your stools. That's because at least half the weight of faeces is bacteria. Let me just repeat that for those of you who've just whispered, "No way". At least half of what you dump into the loo whilst reading the morning newspaper is made up of bacteria. That's dry weight by the way – after all the water is extracted – because it's a highly accurate, comparable and reproducible measure. Wet weight, au naturel, so to speak, the bacterial content is more like 80%, because bacteria, just like us, are mainly water. Similarly, next time you pass wind, blame the bugs. Yes, folks, each of us own a personal biodigester, actively munching away at our leftovers and producing fresh water, methane gas (the flammable one), hydrogen sulphide gas (the smelly one), essential fatty acids, vitamins, and fertilizer as a by-product. It's called the colon. Townies amongst you won't immediately grasp this comparison, but those who live in areas without mains drainage will get it. Poison the biodigester tank buried in your back garden with toilet cleaner capable of killing 99% of all known germs and you're asking for malodorous trouble. Poison your colonic bacteria with antibiotics and the "May cause diarrhoea" warning in the drug information sheet takes on a whole new meaning. Out of interest, old countrymen used to refresh and invigorate the bacteria in their septic tanks by chucking in a dead rabbit or two every spring: fresh food, and an inoculation of all sorts of new bugs from the colon of a different species, does it the world of good.

Some foodstuffs even bacteria find indigestible, notably spices. The heat of chilli peppers (capsicums) is due to the chemical capsaicin, which is completely unaffected by anything our digestive system can throw at it. That's the reason a severely hot curry is called a "ring-stinger". Similarly, castor oil is unchanged, but makes things slip along more easily.

The colon works because it is home to an unfathomably huge microbial ecosystem, which has been compared to the fragile complexity of a rain forest or coral reef. And it now seems increasingly likely the equilibrium of this internal world is crucial not only to our physical health, but to our mental well-being as well. After all, evolution dictates there must be a beneficial reason we've carried and nurtured these, or similar microbes, for millions of years – yet scientists have only recently focused on this synergism. Our colonic ecosystem is presently a right-on trendy subject, as is the word "microbiome", a collective term for all the microbes living on and in us. Advertising companies seem to be using it at every possible opportunity. You can now buy shower gel which is "kind to the skin microbiome", whatever that means. Perhaps it's kinder not to wash at all. Or maybe there's a marketing opportunity here for rabbits: after showering, dry off with a rabbit to reinvigorate your skin microbiome.

Diseases as diverse as multiple sclerosis, diabetes, obesity and mental illness are being linked to imbalances in the colonic microbiome. Faecal transplantation – trans-poo-sion – to restore the balance, delivered either orally or rectally, is being used to treat a variety of mental problems, and is one of the hottest research topics. I kid you not. But it does put an alternative spin on the expression, "shit for brains".

Nevertheless, so long as all those bacteria stay within the colon, they at least cause us no harm; that tennis-court sized internal lining is impermeable to them. If, however, they manage to get where they don't belong, it's a different story, which is why you hope the kitchen staff in your favourite restaurant wash their hands after visiting the toilet. Food poisoning from *E. coli*, *Strep. faecalis* and a host of other faecal contaminants, has public notoriety specifically because of its source, or sauce, of origin.

Perforation of the colon floods the abdomen directly with liquid faeces and attendant bacteria. Despite modern antibiotics and surgery, faecal peritonitis is seriously deadly. It's mostly seen in elderly patients with perforated diverticular disease (small pouches forming in the colon) but a bullet, stab wound, or leaking surgical procedure achieves the same result; overwhelming infection and septicaemia. And when the belly is opened for the inevitable operation, the smell is so eye-wateringly awful it can clear an individual theatre or an entire operating suite of non-essential staff. Hell hath no stench as putrid as faecal peritonitis. It pervades the pores of your skin, your underwear, your hair, and your memory.

But let's get back to Wee Willie.

To be savagely truthful, no one has a clue what causes UC, otherwise it would be a curable inconvenience rather than a life-threatening condition. Varied theories abound, most revolving around auto-immune disease, whereby the body's own defence mechanism is the culprit, attacking perfectly healthy tissue for no known reason. Rheumatoid arthritis, lupus and scleroderma are other examples of diseases where the medical profession invokes "auto-immune" as a pseudo-scientific causality to hide the fact it has no idea. Another term is idiopathic, which roughly translates into "pathetic idiots don't know". Although the cause remains obscure, the symptoms of UC are easy to understand. That all-important impermeable-to-bacteria/permeable-to-water lining becomes inflamed (the -itis in colitis) and drops off to leave ulcers.

I used to explain it to students as follows. Hold out your right arm, it's not quite long enough but it'll do, and imagine it flailed of all the skin, including the skin of the hand and fingers. Then smear it all with shit. It's dripping fluid (water), serum (protein), blood (anaemia), and the shit (bacteria) causes infection. Transfer that image to the colon and you get frequent bloody diarrhoea, dehydration, weight loss, and constant bacterial challenges producing fevers and septicaemia. The result is chronic or acute ill health, and death.

Now let's return to your flailed septic arm, which by now is also dripping pus and causing much grief. Naturally, you consult a doctor who asks how this tragedy came about. Was it scalded, burnt by acid, gnawed by rats as you slept? You reply, 'None of the above.' Some sophisticated blood tests and a biopsy are arranged, but apart from anaemia, raised white count, low protein and a pathologist's report confirming, *"Inflammation and infection of right arm. There is no skin sample in the small biopsy received, which may be significant,"* no light is shed on the matter. 'Mmm ...' the doctor says, scratching his chin, 'are you sure it couldn't be rats? Or mice maybe?' You shake your head, appalled at the thought of rodents in your bedroom. Finally, the diagnosis becomes clear. 'You have idiopathic Ulcerative Armitis,' he says, in a slow sage-like tone. 'I'll treat it with antibiotics coupled with anti-inflammatory drugs and ointments of aspirin and steroids, but I must warn you, it may come to amputation.'

Given the information available, the treatment plan would seem highly appropriate, were it not for a colony of nocturnal flesh-eating termites living undiscovered in your bed post. It seems unlikely the eventual answer to UC will be carnivorous termites, but you get the gist, and my musing may be nearer the truth than any other idea. After all, for hundreds of years Black Death was thought to be caused by evil humours in the air, but was eventually pinned down to a bacterium transmitted by flea bites: *Yersinia pestis*, after Alexandre Yersin who isolated it in 1894.

Willie endured years of appropriate treatment, both orally and rectally, using enemas, but it was time for an amputation. I teed up the anaesthetist and ITU, and Pete Newton was as good as his word, fussing like a mother hen before the surgery and afterwards.

Doing a colectomy is standard stuff for a general surgeon, even one with a special vascular interest. With colitis though, the tissue of the colon can be extremely fragile and is easily torn, thereby spilling liquid faeces all over the otherwise-sterile abdominal cavity. Not good, especially when the patient is immune compromised by steroids, so some gentle care is required.

Once the colon is out and in a bucket, there is a gap between the lower end of the small intestine (the ileum) in the surgeon's left hand, and the upper end of the divided rectum (the rectal stump) in the right. It is possible to restore bowel continuity by sewing the ileum to the rectal stump, but even if all goes well and the ileo-rectal anastomosis heals without leaking, the patient is saddled with continuous diarrhoea and a miserable life. To some extent, the diarrhoea can be reduced by fashioning the ileum into a pouch reservoir of varied complexity at the site of the anastomosis, so defaecation only occurs when the pouch is full. But it's full frequently, so needs frequent evacuation, and pouches are not trouble-free.

As I said to Newton, a pouch was not an option for Willie. He needed something slick and quick, with absolutely no danger of leaking. It was far safer to bring the end of the small intestine out through the abdominal wall and stitch it to the skin as a stoma (mouth), called an ileostomy. The waste from the small bowel then drains into what is popularly known as a "bag", but in polite circles is called a stoma appliance. Having no colon (it's in a bucket by now, remember) to absorb water from this waste fluid causes potential problems with total body fluid balance, but this is easily overcome with a fluid balance chart, sound arithmetic and a good IV line, and the body eventually compensates for absence of the colon.

With the ileostomy done, the rectal stump still remained. What to do with it? To use the flailed arm analogy again, the remaining rectum would amount to about four fingers of diseased tissue. Not enough to cause severe problems, particularly now the river of faeces has been diverted upstream, but troublesome, nonetheless. The rectal stump continues to bleed a little, produces mucus, harbours infection and occasionally needs evacuation (faecal matter, you'll recall, is mainly bacteria). It can be intensively treated locally via the anus, but it was thought easier to bring out the upper end of the rectum onto the abdominal skin as an additional stoma (a so-called mucous fistula) and instil therapy from above. This, of course, leaves the patient with two bags, or at best one bag and an additional messy dressing. Which is preferable for a sixteen-year-old boy: occasional soiled underwear or a permanently soiled dressing on your belly? I voted for the underwear and sewed the rectal stump closed with two layers of good strong sutures. Give it a couple of weeks, and whatever the physicians wanted to shove up his bum (enemas, suppositories, scopes), no surgical harm would come of it. I thought of writing "No Entry for Two Weeks" in felt-tip pen across his buttocks, but settled instead for a big red warning sign on the front of his notes.

In the event, the operation was indeed slick and quick, thanks in large part to the anaesthetist who, forewarned, didn't take an age to get Wee Willie on and off the table. The ITU staff, as ever, were great, using their collective paediatric knowledge to good effect – Will was still a small child, despite his age – and Pete Newton, as he put it, "rescued his patient from the surgeons" back to a medical ward and the umbrella of his continuing care as soon as he could.

Wee Willie was the beginning of a fruitful, though not entirely frictionless, collaboration between the two of us that lasted several years. Until, as a general surgeon with a vascular interest, I negotiated the appointment of an additional general surgeon with a colo-rectal interest to lighten the load. 'Uh?' my colleagues complained, 'General surgery *is* colorectal surgery, isn't it?' 'Afraid not,' I said, 'Not anymore. Now it's a sub-specialty.'

At least three years later, I was walking along one of the many hospital corridors when a tall strapping young man halted me to say hello. I'm of moderate height but no midget, yet I needed to look up – blankly, as it happened – at his face. Patients who you've not a cat in hell's chance of remembering will stop you in the street to say, 'thanks.' This one was no different, though being a vascular surgeon, if one leg had been considerably shorter than the other, I might have been in with a chance. There's a similar old yarn regarding a proctologist who never recalled any of his patients until after inserting a proctoscope: "Ah, now I remember you. Good morning, Mrs Brown."

'You don't recognise me, do you?' the young man said, his smile broad and delighted.

I conceded with a false grin. 'I'm sorry, but I'm afraid I don't.'

Generally, such an encounter is met with how I did such a good hernia repair, or the ingrowing toenail is much better.

'I'm Wee Willie,' he announced, holding his arms wide in a look-at-me gesture, and then burst out laughing. 'It's good to see you.'

I took a step back to avoid a hug and looked him over. Six foot, broad shoulders, blue-black shadow of close-shaved stubble, and the healthy glow of youth. I checked his features again. He looked like a film star. 'Bloody hell, it is you, isn't it?'

'Large as life and twice as healthy.'

'Twice the size, too. Where've you been, in a growbag?' We were both laughing now. Then, I quizzed him.

He'd just left the OPD after seeing Pete Newton for an annual check-up and was heading for the car park. Pete discharged him from follow-up, so all was well. Although his A levels were delayed a year, Willie was off to Uni that September. A continent pouch operation was still in the pipeline, but he was going to wait until finishing his degree and decide then. There was a girlfriend, a covert question from me – deep pelvic surgery with associated nerve damage can upset a young man's performance – but there were no complaints. After twenty minutes or so, we shook hands and said goodbye.

As he walked away, I reflected on how surgeons, for better or worse, drift into and out of people's lives. Healing someone by sticking a knife into their body, leaving them scarred for life, physically and possibly mentally, is on the face of it, perverse. Yet when there is no alternative other than death or continued suffering, patients willingly submit. Wee Willie had undergone what must be the most primitive operation, an amputation. Not of a limb, but of his colon. His disability was a stoma bag rather than crutches or a prosthesis. Yet his health and his life were transformed.

Finally relieved of the need to devote most of its energy to support a rotten festering colon, his infantile body went into overdrive. And at astonishing speed, he had grown into a man.

Another colorectal patient I remember fondly was a forty-two-year-old man with Down's syndrome called Martin. He may have been another of Pete Newton's – either that or his GP referred him directly to me – but one way or another he ended up in my outpatient clinic alongside his older brother. The parents were either dead or infirm because Martin lived with his brother, who clearly doted on him. In common with most Down's syndrome adults, he was short and rather heavy with an honest and loving demeanour. A white open-necked shirt beneath a smart sports jacket made him look quite the gentleman. Having read the referral letter, I already knew the problem, but asked anyway.

'Constipation and incontinence,' he blurted loudly, without a hint of embarrassment.

We chatted for several minutes, with Martin's brother filling any gaps. The constipation was a lifelong problem, controlled and relieved by diet and various laxatives, but in more recent years he required regular enemas and the occasional manual evacuation. The situation had gradually worsened until now: permanent faecal impaction (an over-stuffed rectum) with nothing shifting naturally, coupled with continuous bypassing of uncontrollable diarrhoea requiring rubber incontinence pants. Saddest of all, he felt his supermarket job, pretty much his raison d'etre, was in jeopardy because of too many bad days when he couldn't risk going to work.

I asked Martin to step into the examination room. With him gone and being prepared by a nurse for a rectal exam, I took the opportunity to speak alone with the brother. It was a tale of dozens of doctors, dozens of treatments, dozens of temporary remissions followed by inevitable relapses. Martin was normally stoical, but the last year or two robbed him of his dignity and he'd become miserable and depressed. 'I'm losing my wonderful happy-go-lucky brother.'

While all the questioning and examination was going on (Martin was in a right mess; the nurse needed to put on a gown and get busy with lots of soap and water), I'd been doing some hard thinking. Cynics might say that's an unusual characteristic in a surgeon, but nevertheless I was willing to put a bet on the underlying problem being Hirschsprung's disease. Commonly associated with Down's syndrome, it's usually diagnosed and surgically treated in early infancy, but Martin was born in the 1950s and it might well have been overlooked. Basically, it's a congenital lack of nerves in the bowel wall: nerves that make the bowel muscle relax to allow the passage of faeces along to the anus. If his lower rectum had a short segment of permanent spasm it would act as a functional, rather than a physical block, yet would be missed by an examining finger or scope. Short segment Hirschsprung's would explain the long history of failed treatments, but my theory was completely immaterial to Martin's urgent problem. He clearly needed something to relieve the symptoms, and investigation and diagnosis of any possible underlying condition was entirely irrelevant. At his age, the treatment would be the same. A simple colostomy would give him a cure, albeit at the cost of a permanent bag, but at least he'd be back in control of his life. And if it didn't work out, the colostomy could be closed again, leaving him no worse off.

After Martin was cleaned up, I sat him down alongside his brother and gave them my thoughts. They readily agreed, so I scheduled him for the end of a list the following week.

Doing a colostomy is easy work. The colon is very obliging in this regard, particularly just north of the rectum where it floats about in an S-shape and is termed the sigmoid. Through a two-inch incision in the left lower abdomen, a short loop of colon can be hooked out with a finger, a hole cut into it, and the cut edges of the colon stitched to the edges of the skin incision. For safe measure, a short plastic rod is inserted beneath the loop with the ends of the rod resting on intact skin. The rod prevents the loop of colon falling back into the abdomen and removes any strain on the stitches whilst the construction heals. After a week or so, the rod is slipped out to leave the pink inner lining of the colon healed to the skin in a so-called double-barrelled stoma, akin to peering down the end of a shotgun, like so: OO. The upstream end pushes faeces into a stoma bag; the downstream end leads to the rectum and produces nothing. The procedure took about thirty minutes, but while Martin was still anaesthetised, I had my registrar to do a manual rectal evacuation. It's a messy job – often accomplished with the aid of a sterile dessert spoon and scented mask – but someone needed to do it, and it's character building. That took another ten minutes and filled half a bucket.

Two weeks later, Martin and his brother were back in the OPD for a follow-up appointment. He was a completely different guy. Hugely excited and happy, he gave me a massive bear hug, pinning my arms down, with the side of his head on my chest, 'Thank you. Thank you for making me human again.'

Now that you're fully familiar with colorectal terminology, I'll tell you about a nun. Nudging eighty and admitted as an emergency from a local convent, she'd spent the major part of her life teaching in the adjoining girls' school. Sat in a bedside armchair and dressed in full habit when I first saw her, she was bathed in golden winter sunshine pouring through the nearby floor-to-ceiling window on the second-floor ward. Outside, the surrounding countryside still sheltered remnants of recent snow in the shadowed depths of ploughed fields and hedgerows. The black/white comparison was stark, which is one of the reasons I remember her so well. Despite her pale face and the IV drip in her arm infusing blood, she appeared serene, hands resting palms upward in her lap, eyes closed in a deep sleep.

It was an early morning ward round with the team. A quick dash before theatres screamed for my presence, before the anaesthetist refused to start until seeing the whites of my eyes. The houseman relayed the history.

'Seventy-eight, admitted by the physicians a few days ago because she was breathless with an iron deficiency anaemia, a haemoglobin of seven and a history of supposed bleeding piles for six months. On rectal examination, she has a malignant-feeling growth at the fingertip, so they bounced her onto us yesterday. I haven't personally repeated the rectal because she'll need a biopsy at some stage. In the meantime, she's getting a four-unit transfusion and I've ordered an ultrasound, mainly to check the liver for mets.'

'The physicians did a rectal?' I could hardly believe my ears.

Mandy smiled at my incredulous tone. She'd been my houseman for five months and would be leaving at the end of January for a medical SHO job. A fine young doctor hoping to pursue a career in medicine rather than surgery, she was savvy enough to understand the good-natured jibe. Physicians generally shy away from such intrusive examination, ignoring the long-proven truth that if you don't put your finger in it, eventually you'll put your foot in it. Indeed, somebody already had: telling a patient that bleeding on defaecation is probably due to piles is unforgivable without first excluding a rectal or colon cancer. But then again, it's not every day one needs to do an intimate examination on a nun.

'Well, it did take them some time to get around to it. She was admitted by the gastro team and Doctor Newton did it on his ward round.'

'Ah, that explains it. The good Doctor Newton would never omit a rectal exam. Now then, when she wakes up can we get her down to my clinic first thing this afternoon? I'll 'scope her there and do the biopsy. Once we get the result, we'll decide what to do.'

My examination confirmed a malignant ulcer about an inch above her anal sphincter. The pathologists reported the small biopsy as cancer of the rectum, well-differentiated and low grade, meaning the cancer cells were not highly aggressive and alien looking (undifferentiated, high grade), but still recognisable as rectal tissue, and therefore likely to be slow growing. Nevertheless, without treatment the cancer would continue to bleed and eventually block the rectum, as well as invading surrounding structures such as the vagina in front and the bone of the sacrum behind. Not a nice way to die, whatever your religion.

Anywhere else in the large bowel, a cancer can be removed together with a good few inches of colon on either side as a safety margin, and the two ends of healthy bowel joined together to restore continuity. But with an anatomically "low" cancer which occurs just above the anus, there's no margin of safety which doesn't include the anus itself. The operation requires an abdominal incision together with one in the perineum to remove the rectum and anus en bloc. Called, naturally enough, an abdomino-perineal excision of rectum, it's usually done by two surgeons working together, one from inside the abdomen above, the other working between the legs on the perineum below, making it a synchronous combined procedure. Since all those words are too long to fit on a standard typed operating list, the acronym SCAPER is used. The perineal part is usually done by the registrar, while the boss works in the belly.

To a layman it probably sounds like unadulterated butchery, and as a student I thought the same, but a SCAPER is a brilliantly good operation. The patient gets an "end" colostomy (single, not double-barrelled as in Martin's case, previously) in the left lower abdomen, but because there's no anastomosis, there's no danger of a leak causing deadly faecal peritonitis, and as far as is possible, the local cancer is completely removed with a wide margin. As in every operation, there are a few technical niceties which need to be observed – taking care of the ureters, for example – but generally it's an all-round successful procedure, given a patient with moderate fitness.

Despite her age, Sister Mary Francis was one such. Her pre-operative morning check and chat were with the nearest thing to blood relatives sitting at her bedside: Mother Superior, a woman old enough to be her daughter, and the local priest, young enough and frightened enough to be her grandson. By then, she wore the usual patient attire, a modest plain nightdress buttoned to the chin, albeit with a short white wimple adorning her head and cheeks. With a now normal haemoglobin of 15 and a clear liver ultrasound scan, she understood the need for surgery and a vice-free life meant she was fit enough to take it. Listed for two o'clock that afternoon, she signed the consent form with calm assurance, trusting her fate completely to God. Or so I thought.

'I have a present for you.' Businesslike, she reached into the bedside locker and handed me a wooden crucifix, nine inches high with Christ depicted in soft spelter and a plinth of darker wood at the base, so as to stand unsupported on a mantelpiece, a desk, or possibly a small altar. Feeling uneasy regarding the religious artefact, and imagining I would somehow be robbing the convent of a precious trinket, I made to respectfully pass it back to her. 'It's lovely Sister, but the time for gifts is after the operation when you're fully recovered and well again, not before.'

With a gentle smile, both her palms pushed it back into my chest, but her cold eyes fixed mine with a hard determination, 'That's exactly why I wish you to take it now. *Before* you operate on me.' Her reply caused a chuckle of amusement amongst the onlookers, but only I felt the dread weight and responsibility of the talismanic offering.

That simple crucifix gathered dust on a windowsill or shelf of my hospital office for twenty years or more. I tried giving it away but there were never any takers. Chucking it in the bin seemed irreverent and possibly way too risky. Would such an act anger a deity? What punishment would befall me? So I left it sitting there, daily mocking the infidel atheist in me for a good part of my life. It eventually vanished, probably during one of the many office changeovers it and I endured. Or perhaps it was left behind when I retired. Whatever – it's now gone, with no stain on my conscience. But it served its purpose: I'll never forget the nun.

In the event, her operation and recovery went without a hitch and she too disappeared, back to the convent where the other nuns cared for her, in all likelihood until she died of old age. The reason I know this is because of a man called Dukes, who is the real hero of this tale. But before I tell you about him, a quick lesson on how a cancer spreads is required.

Cancer is so called because Hippocrates likened such abnormal growths – with their claw-like intrusions into surrounding healthy tissue – to a crab (Greek: *carcinos*). Two-and-a-half thousand years later, we still employ the same word and imagery, though the much later use of the Latin term malignancy (malign, malevolent, malicious) is now interchangeable and probably conveys a richer description of the condition. By way of demonstration, I confess to being crabby most mornings, but only rarely am I ever truly malignant.

So, firstly, the very word cancer informs us it spreads locally by direct invasion. Second, it also infiltrates the fine cobweb of lymphatic vessels which permeate all healthy tissue, and lodges in local lymph nodes, often called glands, near to the primary growth. Third, the bloodstream can carry cancerous cells anywhere around the body where they may seed and grow in places far removed from the primary site (secondaries, metastases or mets). And finally, some cancers shed cells into a body cavity such as the abdomen or chest where they take root, grow as multiple seedlings and produce cancerous effusions of fluid. Sadly, a common example of this type of spread is ovarian cancer, which often presents initially with the swollen fluid-filled belly of malignant ascites.

Now, we can return to Cuthbert Esquire Dukes (1890–1977).

The name Dukes is recognised by every doctor of every nation in the world, and though the likes of psychiatrists and dermatologists may possibly be hard-pushed to remember why he's so famous, as medical students they would have been well versed in the results of his research. But for surgeons and pathologists, Dukes daily shadows their life, guides their thoughts, provides a common language by which to communicate worldwide, and informs the conversation when the need arises to talk seriously to an individual patient about the prognosis of colon or rectal cancer.

Hospital pathologists are very much the unsung heroes of medicine. Hidden away in their labs, examining specimens by eye and under the microscope, they deal with dead tissue and dead bodies: no urgency, no medical or surgical emergencies, no patients, no on-call duty as far as I know, no public recognition of their work, and certainly no glamour. That hype belongs entirely to forensic pathologists, a completely different breed who do the extended training and spawn no end of movies, TV shows and novels. Having done his duty on the frontline in World War 1, Dukes was appointed to St. Marks Hospital in London, a specialist establishment set up to treat diseases of the colon and rectum. He was their first ever pathologist. The year was 1922.

From day one, he would have examined segments of colon and rectum removed by the surgeons from patients with cancer. Each specimen consisted of a length of bowel containing the cancer, together with its mesentery, a sheet of peritoneum that attaches the bowel to the back wall of the abdomen and contains the arteries, veins and lymph nodes supplying that segment of bowel. It was to become his life's work. With help in the form of a grant from the British Empire Cancer Campaign, he meticulously examined and recorded his findings from each and every specimen; the grade of tumour (how aggressive it appears under a microscope), whether it was confined to the bowel or locally spread through it, and the presence of lymph node or vascular invasion in the mesentery. Then, (and this must have been the most difficult part), he tracked down the many thousands of patients for which he had specimens to find out if they were still alive five years after their surgery. After excluding those who died from other causes – not bowel cancer – he compared his pathology findings to their longevity. Dukes then presented his results to the world, "... in a way which will be appreciated and remembered by the surgeon."

To paraphrase his charming scientific prose, read, "surgeons are all so thick I'll keep it as simple as possible."

Below are his results for five-year survival of surgically

treated rectal cancer. Published in 1958, it was a seminal paper that crystallized at least thirty years of intricate research, thousands of patients, and sheer hard slog, into three short lines. I've rounded the percentages for clarity:

Group A (Cancer confined to the bowel): 95% – 5-year survival.
Group B (Cancer spread through bowel): 75% – 5-year survival.
Group C (Cancer spread to lymph nodes): 35% – 5-year survival.

These figures show us that the more widespread a rectal cancer is at the time of surgery, the lower the survival rate is five years down the line. Of course, an advanced cancer such as Group C may inherently be more aggressive and therefore spread rapidly, or conversely, the patient may have ignored the symptoms of a less-aggressive slow-growing cancer for a prolonged time. The statistics alone cannot tell us this, but in a way it's irrelevant; as he said in his paper, they're both sides of the same coin. But for an individual patient undergoing surgery, Dukes' classification of the surgical specimen tells us all we need to know regarding prognosis.

Sister Mary Francis's cancer was Group A, or Dukes A, as it came to be called. That's why I could send her back to the convent knowing she was highly likely to be cancer free and, given her age, would probably stay that way for the rest of her life.

Dukes contributed far more to our knowledge of cancer and other diseases than I've outlined in this micro-biography. Any other man would have had all sorts of honours and accolades heaped upon him by colleagues and the medical community at large. From all accounts they tried hard, but being a religious man, he humbly and persistently refused everything offered, preferring instead to live out his days in quiet anonymity in Wimbledon, London.

Perhaps he felt it enough that his name and work would be quoted for as long as doctors and pathologists talk to each other. For as long as surgeons are forced to cut out bowel cancers and tell their patients whether the pathologist's news is good or bad. For as long as medical students need to know his classification system in order to pass exams.

What better accolade? What better honour?

7

A TEACHING HOSPITAL

After leaving Sussex with the ink still wet on my newly acquired FRCS certificate, I was appointed to a registrar job at The London (now Royal London) Hospital. Situated in the rough, tough, deprived East End district of the city, it's an iconic teaching hospital with a history spanning hundreds of years. Among other luminaries, Frederick Treves once worked there. Played by Anthony Hopkins in the 1980 movie, Treves was the surgeon who championed John Merrick, known as The Elephant Man. The hospital still has Merrick's skeleton.

Walking through the impressive colonnaded entrance for the first time on that early August morning in 1979, I felt a sense of pride. Any number of revered men once climbed these same steps, walked the majestic tiled corridor, and achieved many great things within this splendid institution. After all the years of study, exams and dedicated toil, I'd finally made it to a world-famous teaching hospital. First-class surgeons, leading edge research, latest techniques, superb tuition, and now I was to be a part of it. My intention was to embrace it all and suck it dry.

The job was for two years, rotating through four

different posts, six months apiece, though I'd no idea which specialty would be my first. At the interview they told me the individual posts were yet to be allocated, but my inclination towards vascular was noted and could probably be accommodated. I rang several times over the previous week, but couldn't contact anyone able or willing to tell me where to report for duty. The only logical action was to present myself to the personnel department.

'And where the hell is Mile End hospital?' I asked the woman.

'Back out through the main entrance, turn right and walk along the main road for about twenty minutes. It's in Bancroft Road; you can't miss it. You can get a bus or the Tube, but it's quicker to walk.'

I couldn't be bothered to tell her I was driving. 'And who am I working for?'

She consulted her sheet once more, 'Mr Crowland and Mr Lairdson.'

'Do you have any idea what they do?' Uttered more in hope than expectation.

'Well, they must be surgeons, 'cos they're misters.'

Mile End was a small general hospital annexed to The London and housed in an old Victorian workhouse. If you missed the carved stone set in the wall telling you so, the architecture screamed it out; solid red brick, bow windows with dirty-grey granite arches and cornerstones. It looked cold and oppressive, but the surrounding area was pleasantly village-like, with residential terraced housing, tree-lined streets, a park, a couple of pubs, rows of shops and a thriving cockney community. That year, the *Watership Down* movie was smashing box-office records and Art Garfunkel topping the charts with *Bright Eyes*. A local family butcher used the marketing opportunity to hang his shop window with rows of dead rabbits and a big sign: *You've read the book. Seen the film. Bought the record. Now, eat the cast!* Nearby, a dry-cleaning shop countered the butcher's wit with, *Clothes cleaned while you streak.*

The job turned out to be general and upper GI (gastro-intestinal, or gullets and stomachs), two bosses, me, a houseman, and a one-in-two on-call rota. Similar to the set up I'd just left in Sussex, apart from the more onerous on-call. The other surgical firm was colorectal, a mirror image of mine, with a woman registrar who was my opposite number on the on-call rota. She was pleasant, intelligent and keen, with all the correct qualifications, and, it seemed to me, little experience. Whereas I'd bitten the bullet as a junior registrar for two years, she'd been a senior house officer, one grade below me, so it was her first post in the firing line, where responsible decision-making and independent operating are required. She seemed hesitant about both, so I ended up watching her back and helping out a lot. It would have been fine if I lived on-site – guiding the underling was an integral role in my previous job – but inner-city hospitals don't have accommodation. I was living in a grotty rented flat in north London and getting back extremely late on my nights off.

With regards to the routine work, I spent much of the

six months looking at the back of Crowland's head as he did list after list of rigid oesophagoscopies (gullet scoping) with eighteen inches of stainless-steel tube, an outdated procedure, akin to sword swallowing, and about as dangerous. Flexible fibre-optic scopes were readily available even back then, but he maintained they weren't as good for dealing with strictures. Reluctantly, and at my insistence, he did teach me how to do it, a skill I only ever used once in my whole career, on a two-year-old who'd swallowed his mother's Canadian Maple Leaf earring while she was rocking him to sleep, head on shoulder. The child gulped it down straight from his mum's earlobe and the chest X-ray showed the sharp points had it embedded it in the mid-oesophagus. The tiny paediatric fibre-optic scopes at that time didn't have a channel for a flexible grabber, so I was forced to use a rigid one.

The only other thing Crowland taught me was how to run a diary waiting list. Rather than a TCI (To Come In) form being dumped into a filing cabinet for pot-luck extraction at some unspecified time in the future, all his patients were given a mutually agreed date for their operation at the out-patient clinic appointment. This meant they could plan their lives accordingly around a fixed day, and his planned lists didn't suffer from no-show absentees. For me it was a completely novel system that worked efficiently, and when the time came, I used it for twenty-five years. Other than that, the callow youth in me could find no redeeming features in the cold fish. Early on in my tenure I asked if he fancied an end-of-day pint at the local pub. In a holier-than-thou tone he announced, 'I never ... ever ... drink beer.'

Whilst I could just about cope with Crowland's strange character, my other consultant actively loathed him, and others of his ilk. Lairdson was the antithesis of Crowland, a brash loud northerner, fiercely intelligent, bluntly open and honest, he'd arrived at The London from Manchester a year or two before me. Assisting him to operate was a joy. Swift gentle hands coupled with common sense belied his heavy build and history of semi-professional rugby league playing, which by rights should have made him an orthopod. He knew what to do, how to do it, when or when not to do it, did it well, and did it quick. Watching and assisting him was an education in itself, but he often passed the knife to me, directing, instructing, encouraging, and, as an additional commendation, he liked a beer.

'What the fuck're you doin' 'ere'?' He questioned me on our second or third evening in the pub.

'What do you mean, "Here?"'

'Here, at The London?'

'It's a London teaching hospital, one of the best. I'm here to learn more – feather in my cap, looks good on the CV, all that stuff.'

'They're all wankers. Haven't you realised that yet?'

I thought it might be the beer talking, but we'd only made a slight impression on our second pint. Or perhaps he had a chip on his shoulder about something beyond my ken. Either way, my answer was neutral and politically correct,

'I've only worked for two of you so far, so it's a bit early for an opinion on the whole surgical department.'

'You'll learn.'

And learn I did. More than once I had reason to recall prescient advice given to me by a former boss. 'During your training you'll inevitably work for a poor consultant or two. Try to remember you're still learning something, even if it's how not to do it.'

Many years ago, long before anyone had the bright idea of regular audit and appraisal, a national newspaper ran the headline, "HALF OF ALL SURGEONS BELOW AVERAGE", which grabbed the public interest for all the wrong reasons. It was, of course, a statement of mathematical fact but there was no object, as in half of all humans are below average size, height, weight, intelligence, skill. As such, both the headline and story were derided, but it was perhaps the first public foray into the ongoing and often vexed debate regarding surgical outcomes. And therein lies not the problem perhaps, but the uniqueness of surgery. It is a completely transparent and easily audited endeavour.

Poor pilots will tend to kill themselves long before they get to teach others or carry commercial passengers. Poor physicians can always blame the medicine and try another, though since many have become interventionalists with scopes and heart catheters, they too have endured increasing scrutiny. Unlike whatever goes on behind the closed door of the cockpit or consulting room, surgery is always done under the watchful and judgemental gaze of others – it's called an operating *theatre* for good reason. And surgeons are easily compared using all sorts of parameters: death rates, recurrent hernia/cancer/aneurysm/ulcer/varicose vein rates, numbers of operations per list, length of time taken, ugliness of scars, degree of hand tremor, glove size, neatness of stitches and countless others. You think of it and I absolutely guarantee it's been measured. But physical and/or numerical markers, though easy to chart and compare, are never the whole story. The most skilled surgeon with the steadiest hands will be no better than a butcher if he makes poor decisions, and as far as I know, decision-making is an abstract thought process. Sure, you can study the form, understand the odds, play the percentages, but it often comes down to that gut feeling, the hunch to place a bet, and hunches are unquantifiable. Like gamblers, half of all surgeons will statistically make better decisions than the other half.

Does the patient need this or that operation? Will he survive it? Can I do it? Should I do it now, or wait? Should I refer it elsewhere? If it goes badly, can I live with myself? Is the other surgeon better/worse than me? Such questions are even more acutely barbed in private practice or fee-paying health systems, where the answers can affect one's ability to pay the mortgage or put food on the table. In this regard, one's own moral compass should be enough to keep you on the straight and narrow. Failing that, the opprobrium of one's peers makes an excellent straitjacket. And finally, a surgeon performs in front of an audience in theatre, so his decisions, skill, honesty and integrity are set out for all to see. How then, does it ever go wrong?

Along with a half dozen of my contemporaries, I once spent a week in southern France at a specialist vascular hospital. The surgeons and support staff did nothing else, saw nothing else, treated nothing else but patients with arterial disease – furred-up arteries and aneurysms. It was a centre of excellence. We were all based in London, all vascular senior registrars, all invited as guests to observe and to learn. We saw dozens of complex, even heroic, vascular procedures, attended lectures promoting their virtuosity, were shown wonderful statistics as proof, and were wined and dined like royalty. At the end of the week, before flying back to Heathrow, we held our own private debrief in a cheap local bar. Our impression was unanimous: none of the operations we witnessed were necessary. This was a bunch of guys who were happy to rip each other's research to bits in open scientific meetings, the cream of the London circuit with egos as solid and deep-rooted as nuclear bunkers, yet we all agreed. The trip was an exposition in navel-gazing.

With nothing other than vascular surgery to do, and presumably no other source of income, the whole hospital had either knowingly, or most likely blindly, drifted from the sublime to the ridiculous. The surgeons were spectacularly skilled, yet the whole set-up was an exercise in what's extremely possible, instead of what's conservatively advisable. It's a classic error: "I have an operation, you have a condition, therefore the two must come together," regardless of common sense. They didn't treat patients, they corrected dodgy plumbing as shown on an X-ray. Up to a point, that's almost forgivable, but many operations were on elderly people well beyond their best-before date, who could probably function adequately well on supportive medical therapy, without the need for massive, potentially dangerous, surgery. Yet from the senior surgeon down to the lowliest waitress in the swanky hospital restaurant, everyone honestly and openly thought they were doing good deeds, when in practice, they were suffering from institutional isolation and self-delusion.

General surgery at The London during my time there, seemed to me to be mired in a similar complacency. I was expecting wall-to-wall excellence, but compared to my previous job, found little to spur my youthful enthusiasm. One consultant was possibly the slowest surgeon I've ever witnessed, a sure sign of someone with no idea what they're doing or has been trained in the States, a country that in my experience, produces highly knowledgeable surgeons who operate at a glacial pace. On a personal level I liked the man, he was a good diagnostic clinician and very popular among the staff and students, yet I wouldn't have let him operate on me.

A woman surgeon appeared to sit in the theatre coffee room all day, dressed in greens, chatting to whoever would keep her company, and chain-smoking Dunhill's while her juniors did all the operating. She was however very generous with her cigarettes, though they were an acquired taste. Somehow perfume must have spilled into her handbag, leaving every smoke laced with Chanel No.5.

During my six months of cardio-thoracic surgery, the senior registrar finished his training and became eligible to apply for a consultant post elsewhere. When he was offered and accepted the prestigious job he craved, the whole unit was ecstatic. An excellent surgeon, a thoroughly nice guy and a generous teacher, we all felt he thoroughly deserved such good fortune. His new post was due to start in a few months, so in the meantime he would stay on with us. But when the soon-to-be employers did due diligence on his credentials, they discovered he had never passed the FRCS exam. Somehow this information filtered back to the unit, whereupon he vanished overnight, and as far as I know, was never seen or contacted again. He must have been duping The London and other hospitals for years. No doubt, a lot of red faces in more than one HR department pointed accusing fingers at each other, but the whole issue quietly faded away.

On one occasion, when I was the on-call general surgical registrar for the weekend, and doing a Saturday morning mooch around the wards looking for potential trouble, I came across a young woman in a side room. She was twenty-two, with a saline drip in one arm, and a naso-gastric tube draining dark brown fluid into a plastic bag cradled on the floor. The fluid was brown rather than the usual bile-stained green because of bacterial colonisation, a sure sign of prolonged gut obstruction. The name over her bed indicated she was one of the Professor's patients, and therefore a possible complex case such as Crohn's disease with multiple gut strictures. But perusal of the suspiciously thin notes told me otherwise.

She was being treated for presumed adhesive obstruction, secondary to an appendix operation aged fifteen, and the ward sister told me she had been on a "drip and suck" regime for at least a week. The abdominal X-ray showed telltale loops of distended small bowel with the tip of the naso-gastric tube in the stomach, where it should be, but the date on the film was nine days prior. Ding! Ordinarily, at least in my world, she would have been given a few days of conservative treatment (nil-by-mouth with a drip for hydration, and suck – the naso-gastric tube – to deflate the gut) and booked for surgery if there was no resolution. When I checked, her belly was swollen with a neat little appendix scar, but there was no pain, a good thing. Pain would indicate strangulation of a segment of bowel, or worse, a perforation. *This is ridiculous: she should have been sorted ages ago. Nine days without food, she'll have no strength left in her.* Repeat X-rays confirmed there was no improvement. If anything, the bowel was even more distended.

'You need an operation,' I told her.

'At last. Thank you.'

Any abdominal surgery will produce adhesions. Basically, they're flimsy wisps of scar tissue sticking loops of intestine together, or sticking them to the inside scar of the original incision. Generally, they cause no problems, but occasionally a loop of bowel kinks or twists around an adhesion and then obstructs, just like the garden hose which suddenly dries up as you reach the furthest flower bed, and you need to walk back across the lawn to undo a sharp kink. If you're a scientific, experimental type of gardener, you might venture to turn off the tap and disconnect the hose before tackling the kink, and you might then find the reduced water pressure has allowed the hose to relax and undo itself, a similar process to the nil-by-mouth and "suck" part of the conservative treatment. But the girl's tap had been turned off and the hose disconnected for nine days. It was time for definitive treatment.

I don't remember the specifics of her surgery, but I did it that Saturday afternoon, following the obstructed distended small intestine down to the junction with the empty collapsed part, snipping the troublesome adhesions in between, freeing up the kink, and watching the upper bowel deflate as it poured fluid into the lower collapsed segment. Easy, simple, curative, and I'd done the common registrar-grade operation dozens of times. On my Sunday morning mooch she was sitting out of bed, the naso-gastric aspirate was green and reduced in volume, and her belly was flat. Within a day or two, she'd be farting like a trooper and shitting for Britain. Then, she could eat and drink. Job done.

By nine the following morning, Monday, I was no longer on call, but still faced a routine workday to get through before I could go home, collapse into my own bed, and catch up on some sleep. The bleep squawked at around eleven-thirty and I was summoned by a secretary to the professorial unit on the top floor of the hospital, 'Mr Bloggs wishes to speak to you.' With no idea who he was – I honestly don't recall his real name – or what the call was about, I forced my leaden legs up beautiful curved mahogany staircases, followed by functional ugly ones, and made my way to the slanted eaves of the garret. On finally reaching the dismal wooden corridor, I was met by a tall blond guy wearing a clean white coat over a dated floral shirt and matching tie. A few years older than me, I recognised him as one of the surgeons I'd seen in the theatre suite, and though we'd never spoken or been introduced, he struck me as a typical public-school-gone-wrong type: an overly loud, self-important plummy accent, with unbidden yet frequently voiced ear-cringing opinions on anything and everything. The name-tag on his lapel allowed me to finally put a name to the face, "Mr Bloggs, Lecturer in Surgery", which meant he was a grade above me, a senior registrar by another name, and an academic in the professorial unit.

In turn, he studied my badge, 'Ah, you're here.'

The penny finally dropped. It was about the girl. I was there to be thanked for saving the collective professorial backside. 'Yeah, you wanted to speak to me.'

'You operated on my patient.'

'If you're talking about that obstructed girl, then yes, I did, but the Professor's name was above her bed. If she belonged to you as well, then I'm guilty on both counts.' I smiled at my own wit, expecting a similar response. Patients only ever "belong to" consultants or professors, never juniors.

He was unmoved. 'I was going to do her today, this morning in fact.'

'Well, there's no mention of that in the notes. I thought she needed doing, so got on with it. Looks like I saved you the job.'

'You had no right to operate on her.'

'What?'

'I said, you had no right to operate on her.'

'Yeah, I heard you the first time. Who, exactly, *did* have the right to operate on her?'

'Me, of course.'

The conversation was going way beyond what I expected. Exhausted and irritable, I wanted whatever this was about to go away, so I stayed reasonably civil. 'Look, if I jumped the gun on you, then I'm sorry, but I was the on-call registrar and she needed doing. We both know it. If you wanted to exercise your right, as you put it, you should have done so last week, rather than wait till toda–'

'How dare you criticise me!' He'd suddenly gone really narky.

'Hey, hold on, I wasn't having a go. I'm sure there are perfectly good reasons she couldn't be done earlier. Other emergencies, no list time, all that crappy stuff we all have to deal with. All I know is, I wouldn't have left it so long.'

'Listen to yourself, you're doing it again!' He looked at me like shit on his shoe. The volume of our voices was gradually increasing, mine from incredulity, his from affected insult. Then, he bent forward, leaning over to hiss into my face, 'I find your behaviour quite intolerable. In fact, I'm minded to discuss it with the professor.'

At that, I lost it, well and truly. Like an immature school

prefect, this chinless streak of piss was actually trying to intimidate me. Now, it was my turn to lean into his face, my voice a low grumble, the first movement of an avalanche. 'Well, chum, I think that's a fucking brilliant idea. Let's do it right now shall we? Let's both go and see the headmaster and discuss my behaviour. While we're at it, we can discuss how badly you were treating that girl. I'm all for it. That's his door at the end of the corridor isn't it, the one with Professor written on it? C'MON, LET'S GO.' I started striding the twenty yards or so, determined to hammer on the door and put an end to the farce. There was work to do on the wards and an afternoon list to get ready.

Practically sprinting to block my path, and putting both palms up as if to physically halt me, he whispered, 'He's not in.'

I was so incensed that if he'd touched me, I'd have floored him. Through gritted teeth I snarled, 'Get out of my way ... NOW!'

He backpedalled as I marched forward, 'I've told you, he's not in.'

'Well, let's knock, just in case, shall we?'

By now, we were standing toe-to-toe in front of his boss's office, but I didn't need to knock. The door was suddenly flung open and the man himself stood there in shirtsleeves, tie loose at his open collar, one hand cradling a Dictaphone, the other on the doorknob. He was not a happy bunny. 'Whatever it is you two are arguing about, TAKE IT ELSEWHERE.'

I almost laughed out loud, but managed to suppress it.

Instead I smirked, long and slow, first at the prefect, then at his boss, and turned for the exit. As I'd been warned, the place really was full of wankers, and most of them were in the academic unit.

Overall, though, I enjoyed The London job. I didn't learn any more general surgery, but had lots of additional practice, and Lairdson in particular, helped to fine-tune my technique and boost my confidence by putting increasingly complex work on my list. Sadly, I didn't get to do the vascular firm – a few of the other registrars were also keen, so it ended up being a name-out-of-a-hat raffle – though my disappointment was tempered by six months cardio-thoracic surgery. That taught me how to open a chest, operate on lungs, do coronary bypasses, put someone on a heart-lung perfusion machine, and introduced me to the miraculous, instantaneous life-changing cure of mitral valve replacements. Indeed, the job was so enjoyable and rewarding I briefly considered changing my career path, but coronary bypass surgery, much of the work, has to be the most numbingly tedious procedure in existence. As luck would have it, within a few years the operation (CABG: cabbage; coronary artery bypass grafting) was largely superseded by cardiologists with balloon catheters and stents, and the national need to employ more cardiac surgeons evaporated overnight.

The cardio-thoracic theatre boasted one completely novel feature, a wired-in stereo system with an eight-track tape player. I'd never encountered music in any operating theatre before, but soon realised it was installed to relieve the boredom of CABGs – music to lose the will to live by. The choice was limited by the small selection of tapes available, but the Beach Boys *Greatest Hits* usually played non-stop on a loop because it offended the fewest ears. One could always tell if an operation was going badly when *Lady Lynda* or *California Girls* came around for a third or fourth time. To this day, I suffer instant drowsiness and glazed eyes whenever I hear their music played. No offence to the Boys, or their fans.

In modern operating theatres it's uncommon not to have background music, though it's generally "easy listening" rather than hard rock or anything serious. Surgeons who insist on classical stuff quickly discover the other theatre staff get very Brahms and Liszt off.

Although general surgery at The London, with a few notable exceptions, was uninspiring, the design and structure of the building never failed to enthral and enchant me. An antiquated porter's lodge ("Good morning, sir.") with a huge message board just inside the main entrance, the ornate windows and decor, the Nightingale wards, the maze of dusty subterranean and attic corridors, stunning plasterwork and staircases ... every day held a new delight. Most of all, the nurses' uniforms were spectacular: calf-length full dresses with puffed shoulders, short sleeves, huge buttons, white collars and crisp white aprons, all topped with a lace cap. The colours ranged from lilac for a student nurse, through deeper hues of blue for increasing seniority; likewise, the lace cap became more ornate with a train at the back. Every qualified nurse also sported a highly decorative silver belt buckle, invariably a graduation present from their father. On high days, holidays and Christmas, the sisters would don long sleeves, stiff white cuffs, an even longer train to the cap, and parade around each other's wards handing out gifts or singing carols. The whole ensemble harked back to the late Victorian and Edwardian era, courtesy of a Norman Hartnell design of 1942, and looked perfect against the historic backdrop of the hospital. Regretfully, it was completely inappropriate for modern nursing and its days were numbered, soon to be replaced by the universally hated sky-blue "J-Cloth" NHS uniform.

Of the four rotation jobs I did, my six months at Queen Elizabeth Children's Hospital, Hackney, another Victorian edifice but decorated throughout with Disney cartoon figures, was the most enriching. The consultant was an energetic firebrand called Margaret Welland, who held a particular, but not exclusive opinion of surgeons at The London: 'Most of those fools couldn't operate themselves out of a wet paper bag. I hope you're not one of them.'

About ten years older than me, and easily the youngest chief I ever worked for, she was driven by a messianic work ethic, a keen intellect, a complete disregard for the standard 24-hour day and was technically superb. Much of her training had been in Australia, which probably explained her forthright and didactic manner – Ozzie surgeons are not renowned for subtleness. As the only paediatric consultant surgeon she was permanently on call, though on occasion a senior lecturer from Great Ormond Street would be shipped-in to allow her a holiday. The whole hospital called her "Aunty Mags", a term of endearment which held no warning regarding her alter ego of fire-breathing dragon when faced with incompetence. I respected and liked her immensely, but always felt she was touched by loneliness, married perforce to the job with little free time for a life outside work.

I was handed an Air-Call roaming bleep and informed I was also on call 24/7, though there was a career paediatric SHO beneath me, with no need to live-in. In practice, this meant I attended out-of-hours for appendixes, twisted testicles and other relatively simple paediatric emergencies, never wandered far from the East End, did a ward round seven days a week, and remained teetotal for much of the time. Complex treatment and diagnostic work was done by the physicians, who also received neonatal surgical emergencies such as intestinal obstruction, diaphragm hernia, tracheo-oesophageal fistula, spina bifida, hydrocephalus and a legion of other rarities. Sick neonates such as these require medical stabilisation and optimisation by paediatricians before any surgeon is involved, so they never bothered me until a decision to operate was made.

Since I've mentioned rarities, I should tell you the paediatricians were obsessed with them, particularly genetic anomalies, for fear of missing one. On ward rounds they would often examine a child and discuss the possibility of an FLK – something I'd never heard of – then run to the office where a huge well-thumbed tome entitled "Congenital Syndromes" resided. In it were black and white photos of babies and infants together with relevant text describing a recognised syndrome with its signs and symptoms. There were many hundreds of illustrated examples, making the whole book resemble a rogue's gallery of Scotland Yard's most wanted list, but full of mugshots of odd-looking little people. 'What about that one?' 'Nah, the ears are different.' 'That one then, those ears look right.' 'Yeah, but the eyes aren't the same and it's got six toes.' Whereupon the whole crew would go back to the cot and take another look. Initially, I thought FLK must be a variant of Klinefelter's syndrome, one of the rarities even I knew about, where boys inherit one or more additional female X chromosomes, making them XXY or XXXY instead of the normal XY. But no, FLK stands for "Funny Looking Kid", not a derogatory term, but a valid observation alerting everyone to a possible underlying condition. These days, a routine genetic screen would give a definitive answer, so the reference book is probably confined to history. Another term I picked up was "Flat Head" syndrome, seen in older children and adults who spent much of their early infancy in an incubator. Being nursed at that young age with the head on one side or the other for prolonged periods, the soft skull and face bones become moulded to the flat surface of the thin mattress. The long-term result is an elongated skull with facial features flattened from side to side, and the ears unusually flat to the head. Now you know, you'll notice it quite regularly.

Ninety percent of elective paediatric general surgery is

groin work; hernias, hydroceles (water on the testicles), high testicles, circumcisions. Miss Welland would do a hernia, for example, in ten minutes, and by the time my six months' post was finished, I could match her technique across the board, a skill I used and taught to trainees until the day I retired. It was a happy time for me: interesting, educationally useful and fun, my colleagues all first-class and totally committed to the children. Mind you, it's almost impossible not to be committed to a child.

Baby mammals with their big eyes, button nose, small features and disproportionate head size are specifically designed to elicit empathic feelings of love and protection in adults of the same species. That's why calendars with photos of kittens, puppies, human babies and other young mammals sell so well, and all the villains in cartoons look like adults with big noses, small eyes and heavy eyebrows, whereas the heroes and heroines appear childlike whatever their supposed age. Humans regard mammalian youngsters as "cute" without realising it's hardwired into our brains. Medics are not immune, but quickly learn sick kids can also go downhill and die with alarming zeal, adding anxiety to the emotional storm. Of course, women and mothers are more attuned to this natural response, but when I first became a father it was a shock to discover the sound of my baby daughter's cries would harpoon my psyche with unbearable discomfort. Thereafter, hearing *any* child crying reproduced the same angst throughout my working life. Although I felt perfectly at ease doing paediatric surgery, the prelude of frightened weeping and screaming as the anaesthetist did his work would have me running out of earshot until the kids were safely asleep and on the operating table.

Working with children is a hazard to health. Kids are a broiling cauldron of viruses, readily passed on to adults with an immune system totally unprepared for the onslaught. For the whole six months, I was never without a snuffle, cold, sore throat, low-grade fever or other ailment, despite becoming an obsessive-compulsive hand washer. The paediatricians laughed and comforted me, saying I would eventually become immune to everything except head lice, but it takes a few years. Teachers voice similar opinions.

Ward rounds, other than the neonatal ward where all the patients occupied incubators, were organised pandemonium and took forever. Unless they were really ill, no child was ever in their bed and needed to be found in the scrum on the floor or in the playroom. One pretty little four-year-old girl, all ginger hair, freckles and green eyes, seemed to me to spend her life strapped into a yellow plastic toy car, being pulled around on a rope by whoever would volunteer. Her screams of delight were enough incentive to take over the rope whenever it was dropped by someone with work to do. I soon learned she was a urology patient with spina bifida, paralysed from the waist down, constant bladder and rectal problems, and a semi-permanent resident. Without the car, her only other forms of locomotion were a wheelchair pushed by an adult, or crawling on her hands and elbows dragging her flaccid legs behind. It broke my heart to watch, so I towed that car around at every opportunity, including ward rounds.

Later in my career, long after I'd turned into a gnarled old man, a vibrant green-eyed young woman with long flame-red hair manoeuvred her wheelchair through the door of my clinic. Yes, I know it's a recurring theme, but what the hell. It was her, with renal failure, needing an arteriovenous shunt in her arm for dialysis. After years of back pressure and infection, her long-suffering kidneys were finally giving up the fight, and along with all her other struggles, she now faced years of haemodialysis. Peritoneal dialysis wasn't an option because of previous bladder surgery – intra-abdominal adhesions and implanted peritoneal catheters don't get on well. I knew it was her because the yard-thick notes held brown faded letters from the by-then defunct Hackney hospital, and the dates and details fitted. She admitted to spending most of her infancy there, even recalled the yellow car with great fondness, then she broke my heart all over again, 'Nah mate, dahn't remember ya a' orl.'

Unlike other branches of medicine, paediatric patients don't just grow older, they grow *up*, into adults. There must be a limit, a line in the sand if you like, when the paediatrician says, "Too old for me," and hands over a long-term charge into the care of adult medical services. Have you ever wondered when that is? No? Well, neither had I. So, I asked. The consultants spoke earnestly of transition planning, the stage of the disease process, availability of adult specialists, patient and parent wishes, secondary school age, mental age, or actual age: 13, 16, 18, even 21. It was confusing. More so, because I never saw a patient old enough to vote and drive themselves to a pub, sitting in a kids' clinic waiting to be seen by a consultant paediatrician. Eventually, I got the lowdown from the paediatric junior doctors:

'It's pubes. Once they grow pubic hair, they're out.'

Obvious really. Staring you in the face.

———

Towards the end of my time at The London I needed to find a research post. Getting yet another degree was, and probably still is an imperative. The one to go for was Master of Surgery (MS, or MChir if you're posh) and the ad pages of the BMJ was where to find it. I wanted something to do with vascular surgery, but there were few to choose from, and all in academic units. My poor regard for academic surgeons meant I wasn't relishing the task. I did get an interview in Birmingham for a post requiring dog and pig vivisection – something I wasn't too keen on – but when the Prof asked me if I would be able to care for the animals post-op, and I told him truthfully I wouldn't have a clue how to do it, it was clear the job wasn't suited to me. The rejection letter confirmed it.

While the hunt for the salvation of my future career continued, I happened to attend an evening meeting at the College of Surgeons. It was a prestigious Hunterian lecture on Raynaud's Phenomenon, a relatively common problem of inappropriately cold blue hands described by a French physician in the mid-1800s. No one understands the condition, yet it's constantly seen in clinical vascular practice. For completeness, I should also tell you that John Hunter was a surgeon, anatomist and polymath of the 1700s who made his name in London, and to this day is widely revered, particularly by the College.

The lecture was well-attended by old men in suits, though the front seats were occupied by a gaggle of young guys who looked out of place in jeans and jackets (like me, hiding at the back), and many of them had beards and long hair. Afterwards, they were all noisily enjoying themselves in the normally very conservative and hushed bar, most of the old men having disappeared after the medal presentation ceremony. The guy who'd given the excellent lecture, a young surgeon called Aiden Beamish, looked incongruously overdressed in an ultra-smart suit, yet was the centre of their excited attention. I didn't know Aiden from Adam, but wandered over to congratulate him and mix with my kind. Several beers later, I ascertained they were all from a biomedical engineering research unit based in Dulwich, south of the river, and part of King's College Hospital. Much of their research was vascular based, the unit stuffed with post-grad students doing a PhD – which explained all the beards and long hair – and, at any one time, there were two surgeons doing MS work. Surgeons and pure scientists toiled collaboratively in one big, messy, productive, happy family. Looking around at the drunken rowdy gathering, I could well believe it. The only po-faced person in the place was the barman, clearly unhappy at pulling countless pints for young ruffians when his usual custom was the genteel small sherry and G&T brigade.

By pure serendipity I'd discovered the ideal research job for me, complete with equally ideal workmates. 'I've just got my MS, so I'll be pushing off in a month or two,' Aiden explained. 'They'll need another surgeon and you seem just the ticket. What do you think?'

'Sounds right up my street, but I've not seen it advertised yet. Who runs the show? I could write a pre-emptive letter with a CV.'

'Better than that, let me introduce you. That's him at the end of the bar. He's paying for all this, so the least you could do is thank him for buying you a beer.'

He wasn't joking. 'What? The barman told me it was free, but I thought he meant it was on the College. Oh, bloody hell, Aiden, I'm so sorry to have gatecrashed your private celebrations. I had no idea.'

'It's the jeans and jacket; you fit in perfectly.'

It was the first time I met Jack Walters. He was to have a profound effect on my life.

8

VASCULAR SURGERY

George was a splendid old boy in his mid-seventies. Dark blazer, regimental tie, grey trousers with a razor crease, black mirror-shiny shoes, all topped with a Brylcreemed short back and sides. Sitting on the other side of my Thursday morning out-patient desk, legs crossed in an easy self-assured manner, he was trim, lean, and looked fitter than me, almost thirty years his junior. He'd seen and done it all while I was still in nappies and short pants, including Korea and Suez, but never lost the military habit and staunch allegiance to his comrades. I knew all this because the small parachute emblems on his tie piqued my interest, and a patient's history is an important part of any medical consultation. I also understood enough not to press him further. The wistful look in his rheumy eyes told me his attire wasn't the result of bravado or boast, but remembrance. Some people always wear a hidden-in-plain-view memento of a lost life or love, be it a ring, a tie, an old wristwatch, a brooch, or a colour, and pass it off as a personal quirk. George did it for his fallen mates.

'I told my doctor I thought my heart had somehow slipped into my belly. I could feel it pumping away where it shouldn't ought to. She sent me for a scan and next thing I know I'm here in front of you, double-quick, I might add. So, what's to do?' He spoke as if his normal routine was being upset by a minor inconvenience.

George's heart hadn't migrated to his abdomen, though I'd heard his interpretation many times before. The ultrasound scan confirmed the pulsating swelling in his belly was an abdominal aortic aneurysm. And a dangerously large threat to his life.

The single large artery carrying blood away from your heart is called the aorta, the main highway of the arterial system. Every minute, about the time it takes you to sit quietly and read these few sentences, all the blood in your body – that's five litres, eight pints, or a gallon – circulates back to the heart, passes through your lungs to pick up oxygen, and gets pumped out into the aorta again. At about 2cm (just under an inch) in diameter, it's somewhat wider than a garden hose, and arches backwards within the chest before coming to lie next to the spine. Smaller branches coming off the aortic arch sequentially supply high-pressure oxygenated blood to the right and left coronaries of the heart, the right arm, the head and neck via the right and left carotid (Greek for stupefy, because compression or division starves the brain of blood; see also many Tarantino films), and finally a branch to the left arm. Thereafter, the aorta runs south in front of the backbone and pierces the diaphragm to enter the abdomen, where further branches supply blood to the spleen, liver, gut, kidneys and pancreas, until at about the level of the belly button, it forks neatly into two, one branch to each leg.

As you might imagine, like a hosepipe used continuously for fifty years or more, with age the aorta tends to weaken in places and expand. Weak expanded segments are called aneurysms, from the Greek *aneurusma* meaning dilatation. Interestingly, and to digress for a moment, comparative anatomists have suggested the structure of the aorta in different animals – including humans – correlates with the life expectancy of that species. In other words, it seems the thickness and elasticity of the aortic wall has built-in redundancy and is doomed to lose its integrity towards the end of a normal lifespan and become aneurysmal. Of course, like an old hosepipe, an aneurysm can only balloon out so far before it bursts.

The most common place the aorta develops an aneurysm is in the abdomen, just upstream of where it divides into the two leg arteries. Engineers will immediately think of reflected standing pressure waves occurring in pulsatile flow, which may well be contributory. Two in every hundred men over sixty-five will have some degree of aortic swelling in that area on ultrasound scanning, prompting the introduction of national aneurysm screening programmes in this age group. In comparison, women are much less likely to develop an aneurysm (perhaps 1 in 400), so don't get screened. It's undeniably an old man's problem. More so, because it has few, if any, symptoms.

Dropping down dead due to rupture is the most common symptom and happens in 90% of undiagnosed patients if some other problem doesn't kill them first. Of those that reach an operating table alive, half will also die. So overall, the mortality of ruptured abdominal aneurysm is 95%. Up to a hundred years ago or less, drop-down-dead-itis was usually blamed on a heart attack – as were many other conditions, such as a clot on the lungs, massive stroke, brain bleed, poisoning – and the evidence burned or buried according to the corpse's wishes. That's why, depending on your age and regardless of the real cause of his demise, family lore will often have your grandfather or great grandfather, "dropping dead of a heart attack." In any case, it matters not a jot what he died from – unless it was an electric chair or at the end of a rope, in which case you've been told lies – because back then it was more likely than not untreatable, and anyway, dead is ... well, dead, whatever the cause. The point is, at least 2% of all elderly men throughout history had an abdominal aortic aneurysm (AAA or Triple A) and unless some other disease intervened, would have dropped dead due to it rupturing. Without treatment, George would soon be joining them.

His aneurysm was exactly 6.5cm in diameter, over three times the normal size. If it were to rupture, he had a 90% chance of dumping all his circulating blood into his belly within a minute or two. In plumbing terms, this is equivalent to a mains water pipe bursting, the type that throws flagstones and lumps of tarmac into the air and floods the street, leaving homeowners banging their tap and wondering where all the water's gone. Thankfully, a brain starved of blood due to a burst AAA would have only a few sentient seconds to wonder where all the blood's gone, so any awareness of pain and suffering would be mercifully short and replaced by a deep endless sleep. Not a bad way to go.

If you've been paying attention, by now you should be wondering how 10% ever make it to an operating table. This is best understood by returning to the mains water pipe buried deep beneath your feet. Should a leak occur in the topmost section of pipe, the route to street level is straight up with relatively little resistance to the water pressure, and once the flagstones have gone, a tall geyser appears. A disruption in the lowermost deeper section will tend to be more contained by the surrounding subsoil, so the leak is slower and results in a gentle flood rather than a spectacular fountain. The deepest (posterior) part of the abdominal aorta lies against the hard bone of the spine with dense surrounding tissue, whereas the most superficial (anterior) part has a paper-thin sheet of peritoneum. The lesson here is, if you want to go quick and clean, have an anterior rupture. Posterior leaks often produce painful backache and death approaches more sedately, thereby giving surgeons a small time-window in which to act.

At 6.5cm, George's aneurysm had a greater chance of killing him than I did. I knew this because of research, not necessarily mine, but worldwide follow-up of patients with Triple A's, and the results of surgery to treat them. The foremost work in this regard was British. The UK Small Aneurysm Trial (published around 1999) was a credit to UK vascular surgeons as a body, and our national public health system. Before the results of the trial were known, the received wisdom was to operate on any aneurysm above 4.5cm. After the trial, we knew vascular surgeons had been killing more patients – around 4% of all aneurysm repairs – than would have died from rupture. In other words, with small aneurysms it's safer to simply follow them with regular scans rather than operate. At 5.5cm and larger, the tables turn in favour of surgery, which cures more patients of potentially lethal aneurysms, than it kills.

If my seemingly blasé use of the words "kills" and "killing" has affronted your sensibilities, then I apologise. I could have used standard impersonal scientific jargon – "mean thirty-day post-operative mortality of AAA repair is 4%" – and you wouldn't have blinked an eyelid. After all, it's a big operation for a life-threatening condition in elderly patients who often have other medical conditions. But if they die during the surgery or post-op, it isn't the operation that killed them, it's the surgeon. Any surgery-related death is extremely personal for whoever wielded the knife: self-doubt, sleepless nights, guilt, depression, and worse. No surgeon ever plans to avoid ruining the national mean thirty-day mortality statistics. Rather, they aim not to kill the individual patient who's placed his or her life in their bloodied hands. This begins by only operating on patients who are likely to survive.

'Do you mind if I call you George?'

'No, please do, everyone calls me George, or something rude,' he chuckled.

'Well, George, this aneurysm of yours, do you understand anything about it?'

'My son looked it up on his computer. Some sort of swelling on the artery in my stomach which needs a plumbing job? Sounds a tad rum to me.'

He was attempting a joke, but it was no time for humour. 'That's right, George, it is a swelling. But without an operation, I reckon it's got about a one in five chance of bursting and killing you within the next year ...' I paused to gauge his reaction, but he was well ahead of me.

'My son said it was ten percent ... he's a bit of a boffin,' he added, almost apologising for testing me.

'And I'm glad he is. He doesn't happen to be with you, does he?' I was hoping his son was in the waiting room. As far as I'm concerned, when giving bad news, the more the merrier.

'No, he's in Australia.'

'That's a pity. Is anyone with you?'

'No, I'm here on my own.'

'Well please tell your son what I say. It sounds like he's quoting the raw figures for all-comers with a six-centimetre aneur– ... swelling. Yours is a bit bigger than that, you're probably a little older than average, and you're not a big man, so your swelling is relatively larger. It all adds up. Would it sound better at fifteen percent? I suppose when all's said and done, I'm only giving you a reasonable guesstimate based on what we know. And I'd be more than happy to pass you on for a second opinion if you prefer.'

'No need. He looked you up as well. You'll do for me.'

Rather than being flattered, I was more concerned at how the tendrils of the Internet held me within their grasp, even from Australia. Dismissing it as beyond my control, I ploughed on with my usual litany. 'The operation's not without risk, George. Overall, including young fifty-year-olds and old eighty-year-olds, there's about a one in twenty-five chance you won't pull through. It's generally not the surgery itself that's the problem, but afterwards. Heart failure, kidney failure, pneumonia, are all risks. But you look fit enough to me and I'll get a few baseline checks on your heart and lungs first. Are you happy to go ahead?'

'If you say it's for the best, then yes I am.'

'I'm sure it's the right thing to do, but equally, you must understand the risks.'

'The Jerries didn't get me, so I'm sure you won't.' His grin showed the long thin teeth of an old man.

'I'll do my best, George, but I think the sooner you get done, the better.' I began thumbing through the diary looking for a clear list, or I could possibly shuffle a few patients around ...

'How soon is soon?' he said, with a note of concern. He had every right to be worried.

'Frankly, as soon as possible. Give me a minute and I'll sort out a da–'

'I'm getting married on Saturday week, followed by a two-week honeymoon, so it'll have to be after then.'

Stunned, I dropped the diary back on the desk and fixed him with my gaze. He wasn't smiling. 'You're not pulling my leg, are you?

No, he wasn't. His wife died years before. He'd been "stepping out with a close lady friend" for three years. She was also widowed, and neither were getting any younger. Being wed would give them both financial security and companionable happiness in their twilight years. After what I told him regarding the risks of aneurysm surgery – thank you very much – he was more convinced than ever the wedding "must come first". Nor would he cancel the honeymoon, a coach tour of Scotland, and the first time they would be "together day and night". With no defence against such logic, I conceded defeat and we agreed a date for his operation four weeks down the line. Then, I advised him to put his affairs in order ('Already done, Doc.') and not to drive.

Before leaving, he stood up and shook my hand. 'Thanks for being so understanding.'

'She's a lucky lady George, I hope it all goes well. Will I meet her next month when you come in?'

'You certainly will.' A curious smile creased his face. Then, he turned for the door.

A thought suddenly struck me. 'She does know about all this ... doesn't she?'

He looked back and winked, 'Not yet, but soon.' Then, he was gone.

The following afternoon, Friday, I was in yet another clinic when, unusually, the desk phone rang. It was the on-call surgical registrar calling from A&E. She'd already done six months with my firm, so knew the timetable and exactly where to find me. Refreshingly good at her job, I trusted her judgement. Whatever it was about, the call would be necessary and to the point.

'There's an old soldier here with a leaking Triple A. Says he saw you yesterday.'

My heart turned to lead. 'Yeah, I remember him. Is he a goer?' *Meaning: is there enough life left in him to get to theatre?*

'I think so, otherwise I wouldn't have called. He's a bit clapped out, but he's conscious and with us. Theatre's ready and waiting, and there's six units being cross-matched.'

'See you there in five minutes.'

I abandoned the remainder of the outpatients to the registrar, my secretary and the nurses, and took the ever-present medical students with me, three of them. From their excited expressions, it looked like Christmas had arrived early.

By the time I'd changed, donned greens and entered the operating theatre, the patient was already on the table, surrounded by a rugby scrum of anaesthetists, technicians and nurses, all busily concentrating on their individual tasks. Jugular line for venous access and pressure, wrist arterial line for arterial pressure, bladder catheter, oxygen mask, an arm line for additional fluids, ECG electrodes on chest and limbs, an earth plate for the cautery machine, and much more besides. For all this to happen simultaneously, the man was stark naked and spread-eagled, both arms supported on boards, with the table tilted head down to maintain the blood pressure and distend his neck veins for easier cannulation. I pulled down my mask to expose my face and struggled to the head end, needing to confirm for myself it was indeed George, yet all the while hoping by some cosmic chance it was some other poor sod. But it was him. Pale, sweaty, wide awake and terrified.

'Hello George, it's me. Looks like I'm doing you earlier than expected.' The best he could manage in return was a brief grunt from behind the oxygen mask and a nod. I smiled at him, 'Good man, soon have you up and running again.'

You may be wondering why George was still awake. It sounds a bit brutal to be attacking a defenceless naked man in such a manner, and in truth, it is, but it's done with good reason. If you anaesthetise a patient with a leaking AAA, in gasman parlance he'll "crash and burn", meaning whatever blood pressure the physiological response to bleeding – masses of adrenaline, blood vessel constriction, rapid heartbeat – is maintaining, the anaesthetic will knock it out, along with the patient. The blood pressure will then drop to zero and the heart beat itself to death.

The trick is to get all the coconuts lined up and ready (monitoring, surgeon plus assistant and scrub nurse) before the anaesthetic does its best to kill the patient. Getting a clamp on the aorta as soon as possible after the patient is asleep is the priority. Once the bleeding is under control, pour blood in. No point giving it beforehand because within a few heartbeats it's pissed out of the aorta and washing around the abdomen, a waste of an expensive hard-given commodity when other cheaper fluids are available. The conductor in charge of all this pre-op orchestration is the anaesthetist, though every band member knows their individual score. That day, the anaesthetist was also the ITU senior consultant. It boded well. If George made it off the table, he'd be transferred to ITU and be under the gasman's continuing care. As the lead anaesthetist *and* boss of ITU, he had skin in the game. Colin was also punctilious, not necessarily a bad thing in an anaesthetist, but to the degree he could be a pain in the arse.

Several minutes later, George's abdomen was prepped with antiseptic wash, green drapes applied, and I was scrubbed, knife in hand, waiting for the nod. I roped in the sturdiest-looking medical student as second assistant, a big lad who looked as if he wouldn't faint and could hold the bowel out of my way for the next hour or so. He stood to my left. Opposite me was the registrar who started the ball rolling on this one, but had previously assisted me with many elective cases. Next to her was Audrey, my regular aneurysm scrub nurse. The coconuts couldn't have been lined up better. Further to my left, the ITU man whispered from the top end, 'Ready?' I nodded yes. 'Start when I say.' I nodded again. At that he gave the go-ahead to his own registrar who pushed a couple of big syringes full of intravenous agents into the venous line; one drug would anaesthetise, the second paralyse. Colin already held a laryngoscope in his left hand. I watched it bob up and down as he silently counted to ten. 'Go!' he said loudly, before busying himself inserting an endo-tracheal breathing tube and attaching it to the mechanical ventilator.

At that point, in my head, George and the rest of the world ceased to exist. My universe now lay inside this anonymous male belly. It was a simple manual building job, to be done brick by brick, but every single one needed to be laid straight and true. I learned my craft over many years from other bricklayers, some excellent, some less so. The odd slightly crooked brick doesn't make much difference – a living organism has a will to heal itself – but each crooked one can add to others until the whole edifice falls to ruins. Better to make them all straight and true.

The stem to stern midline incision took less than a minute, releasing pints of thin watery blood, most of which escaped the sucker and sloshed to the floor. Audrey handed me the mechanical retractor to hold the wound widely open, then I gathered the slippery bowel, wrapped it in a huge damp swab, pushed the bundle to the right side of the abdomen and placed the student's big hands over the lot. Proudly standing centre stage was the grapefruit-sized aneurysm, gently pulsating and softer than normal due to the low pressure. The back of the abdomen (the retro-peritoneal space) was dark red and tense with clotted blood, typical of a posterior rupture. In places, the flimsy peritoneum had torn under the strain, allowing blood and serum to leak into the abdominal cavity. The imperative was to find a segment of normal aorta above the grapefruit, and clamp it shut. Quickly, but not in haste.

Crossing the aorta from left to right, just where the clamp needs to go, is the thumb-sized left renal vein, on its way to join the even bigger inferior vena cava, running south to north alongside the aorta. And veins, particularly big ones, are frighteningly thin. Once cut or torn, they bleed like absolute bastards and are nigh on impossible to repair with a stitch. Rushed attempts to apply a foot-long aortic clamp, blindly, into that area of anatomy, is almost guaranteed to rip a hole in one or both veins. It's a game-over move I witnessed more than a few times as the assisting registrar. The patient bleeds out in minutes.

Calmly and slowly, using nothing sharper than my fingertips, I cleared a space below the renal vein and on either side of the aorta, until I could feel the hard bone of the spine beneath. Using my fingers as a guide, the blades of the clamp went safely and neatly either side of the normal aorta, just above the start of the aneurysm and just below the renal vein. I squeezed the handle and clamped it shut. The aneurysm stopped pulsating. Success. 'Clamp is on,' I shouted to the top end of the table, hidden behind a screen of green drapes. 'Okay,' came a muffled reply.

Time for a breather. Blood and fresh frozen plasma would now be pouring in. I rested a finger on the aorta just above the clamp and could feel the pulse begin to strengthen. Soon the long clamp would be a bouncing telltale of pulse and pressure. The next stage would involve more bleeding, so I waited, passing time examining the lower part of the aneurysm. Often the weak aneurysmal segment extends into the two leg arteries (the iliacs), a tiresome but easily overcome complexity, though it has the added danger of ripping a hole in one or both iliac veins, another game-over move. But not this time: it would be a straight, rather than a trouser-shaped graft. Without the need for further dissection, I put short clamps on the iliac arteries to stop any back-bleeding from the legs once the aneurysm sac was open. With nothing else to do until the disembodied voice from top end gave me the go-ahead, I took the chance to stand straight, stretching my back and shoulders.

'Do you want Roy on?' Audrey whispered across the table.

'Blimey, I knew something wasn't quite right. It's too quiet isn't it? Yes, of course. We can't do it without Roy, can we? It'll be a disaster.'

'What about him?' She angled her head, indicating our touchy anaesthetist.

'That's his problem. We need Roy.'

Audrey nodded to a student nurse hovering near the CD player in one corner of the theatre. Seconds later, Roy Orbison's greatest hits were playing, beginning with *Only the Lonely*, and we were harmonizing Dum Dum Dum Doo Bee Doo Wah. I don't recall how it began, or why, but Roy was always the talisman for a successful AAA repair. No other music would do. If it was an aneurysm, Roy was the main man.

Inevitably, 'For God's sake, do we have to put up with this racket?' came forth from the top end.

''Fraid so Colin, I simply can't be doing an aneurysm without Roy. Anyway, can I crack on yet? The blood pressure must be good by now.' My left fingertip, resting on the aorta above the clamp, told me it was.

'Yes, get on with it.' He sounded delightfully grumpy.

I sliced open the grapefruit with a knife, lengthwise. The registrar, impressing me with her anticipation, sucked out the half-litre of scarlet blood without instruction, and carried on sucking, quite the bricklayer's mate. 'You've done this before,' I quipped, by way of a compliment. Then, insinuating my fingers between the thin wall of the aneurysm and the thrombus (solid blood clot which develops over years in the turbulence away from the central main stream of blood flow), I extracted a perfect natural cast of the grapefruit's insides, with a 2cm wide channel running through it. After removing the succulent juicy part, all that remained was an almost bisected empty grapefruit skin – the aneurysm sac – the same white pithy colour, with a split along the back left-hand side where the rupture occurred. But it was only a fleeting view, because almost immediately the sac flooded with fresh arterial blood.

I was expecting it, but it needed to be dealt with quickly – blood is too precious to squander. You'll recall I clamped the iliac arteries before opening the sac, to stop back-bleeding from the legs? Well, after the thrombus cast is removed, there are a few other branches that will back-bleed – like a plughole backing up and filling the sink with water from elsewhere – but which can't be clamped, and will piss blood until they're over-sewn and blocked off. This is achieved from within the empty grapefruit, so to speak, closing the origin of each artery with stout sutures. Coming off the front wall of the aneurysm is a big artery to the left colon, and it was hissing blood. That's not a misprint. There's bleeding you can see, bleeding you can feel, as it drips down your legs or soaks up your arms, and bleeding you can hear. The inferior mesenteric artery was hiss, hiss, hissing, with every heartbeat. A good noise, I could over-sew it knowing the colon was getting a decent blood circulation from elsewhere. Along the aneurysm's back wall are three or four paired arteries (eight tiny plugholes) supplying the backbone and spinal cord. They were back-bleeding "briskly", as we say, another indication of a good supply, and were sewn off in the almost certain knowledge it wouldn't cause the extremely rare complication of ischaemic (lack of blood) paralysis from the waist down.

So far, so good. With the aneurysm sac now dry, in the upper part I could see straight into the single tube of normal aorta, whereas the lower part resembled the dangerous end of a side-by-side shotgun, the top of the two iliacs or leg arteries. The gap would be bridged by sewing in a Dacron (known as Terylene in the UK) tube graft. A Terylene shirt or sheet isn't watertight, so a tube of the same material will leak like a colander. But not only is blood thicker than water, it also has its own inbuilt self-sealing mechanism – the clotting system. By soaking the Dacron tube in blood, all the tiny platelets, red cells and clotting factors will get to work, plug the weft and weave of the fabric and render it impermeable. And in leaking aneurysm surgery, there's no shortage of blood. After selecting a 22mm diameter graft I threw it into the pelvis and massaged it in the pooled blood collected there, turning it from virginal white to rose pink.

Fifteen minutes later, using a continuous strong nylon suture and big bites of the needle, the top anastomosis between the Dacron tube and healthy aorta was complete. Finally knotting the suture took seven throws because the knot simply cannot slip or break (game-over), and because seven is a magic number, and every surgeon needs a bit of luck on their side. The aorta/Dacron anastomosis was stress-tested by clutching the free end of the graft closed in my right hand and releasing the aortic clamp with my left. High-pressure arterial blood immediately flooded the synthetic tube which stiffened and pulsed rhythmically. No leaks. Good. By moving the clamp from the aorta and applying it to the middle of the Dacron graft, I freed my hands and continued to test the needlework while getting on with the lower end. If the top end was going to leak within the next ten to fifteen minutes, I'd spot it and deal with it.

The lower anastomosis took another ten minutes or so, but I didn't insert the final stitch because we were approaching a critical phase. 'Colin, I'm almost done here. Are you ready at your end?'

Ever since the aorta was first clamped, perhaps forty-five minutes earlier, the patient's lower body had been starved of arterial blood and life-giving oxygen. All that muscle (buttocks, thighs, calves) and skin would be hungry for it, and consequently full of metabolites (waste chemicals of metabolism) designed to relax and dilate blood vessels enough to satisfy their ravenous appetite. Once the clamp came off, not only would the capacity of the circulation instantly double by reverting to its normal size, but all those stagnant chemicals would get flushed throughout the whole body, causing widespread vessel relaxation. The blood pressure would plummet, and once again, the heart could beat itself to death. Yet another route to crash and burn.

From the anaesthetist's viewpoint, the trick is to infuse more blood and fluids (pre-load) before the clamp is released, thereby staying ahead of the game, yet be prepared to order the surgeon to re-clamp and infuse even more fluid if the pressure drops significantly. His main focus is to keep the pressure within reasonable boundaries, neither too high (risking a stroke) or too low (heart attack).

The surgeon, however, hates static blood. Blood which doesn't flow will clot, and the longer it stands still, the more it clots. The blood in the graft and aorta immediately above the clamp was probably already clotted. Likewise, in the iliacs. That hole I'd left by not putting the final stitch into the lower anastomosis was there to vent any clots that would otherwise be forced down into the legs and cause all sorts of trouble. And once the clamp was off, I wanted it off for good. My main focus was to keep the blood flowing and free from clots.

Colin shouted, 'Two minutes. I'll tell you when.'

Roy was singing, *You Got It*.

While Colin pre-loaded the circulation, I briefly released first one iliac clamp, then the other. As expected, the gentle back-bleeding washed out some clot from both sides, helped on its way by inserting the tip of the sucker into that pre-arranged vent hole.

'Okay, take the clamp off and let's see what the pressure does.'

Working quickly now, I held the cupped palm of my right hand over the vent, and with my left hand, fully opened the clamp. For a second or two, nothing happened. Then, a slug of magenta clot appeared in the vent, slowly extruded to golf-ball size, and exploded with a great shoosh of scarlet. My cupped right hand prevented the subsequent fountain of arterial blood from dousing the overhead lights and everyone around the table. I closed the clamp and briefly released it once more. SHOOSH. No more clots. With the final stitch completed, together with another seven throws on the knot, the clamp was off for good. Putting my right thumb and forefinger either side of the graft told me the pulse rate and gave some idea of the pressure. I yelled, 'Clamp is off.'

At the anaesthetic end, the drapes were lowered, allowing me sight of the blood pressure monitor. It showed a continuous readout from a cannula in the radial artery at the wrist, and the pressure was dropping: 90 ... 80 ... 70 ... 60 ... Between my thumb and forefinger, I squeezed the graft almost, but not completely, shut, surreptitiously allowing some blood to pass in order to prevent any clotting. I could feel it sizzling past my fingertips. The pressure started rising: 60 ... 70 ... 80 ... 90 ... Colin and his registrar pushed more blood. I released. 100 ... 90 ... 80 ... 80 ... Squeeze. More fluids. More blood. Release. 100 ... 100 ... More blood. 110 ... 110 ... 120 ... Then, I finally relaxed. The pre-load had been judged well. Sometimes this waltz could take twenty minutes or more before the pressure stabilised. Removing my fingers from the graft completely,

I shouted, 'Colin, the clamp's off for good. You okay with that?'

'Yep.'

It still wasn't quite finished. I needed to check that the foot pulses, there before the operation started, were still present afterwards. That would tell me no clots were blocking the leg arteries. But being scrubbed, I couldn't do it myself, and foot pulses are notoriously hard to feel if you don't know where to place a fingertip. Audrey asked her student nurse to push back the green drapes to uncover the feet. Both looked pink (good), and both bore the mark of a black felt-tip pen on the instep, put there by me over an hour previously. I asked the student nurse if the marks were pulsating. Hesitantly, she placed a finger on each, 'Ooh ... ooh, yes ... yes, they are!'

After some general housekeeping to mop up spilled blood and fluid within the belly, the empty grapefruit skin was folded over the Dacron graft and stitched in place. This would reinforce both anastomoses and stop loops of gut sticking to the foreign material. I closed the midline incision but left the skin stitch to the registrar and student. After pulling off my gloves and gown, I checked the foot pulses myself, then wrote the operation notes, leaning on the stainless-steel table next to the CD player. Roy was crooning, *It's Over*.

One of the other two observing medical students approached me with the obvious intention of asking a question. She seemed a little nervous and timid, so I pulled down my mask, gave a friendly smile to put her at ease, and mentally prepared myself to answer an erudite searching query on the finer points of aneurysm surgery. 'Hello, how can I help?'

'Who's Roy Orbison?'

Peering into her impossibly young face, I couldn't formulate a satisfactory response. The chasm of years between us was just too wide. And besides, my nicotine and caffeine levels were red-lining. So I pointed towards Colin, 'Ask the anaesthetist, he's the real fan.'

Walking down the theatre corridor towards the coffee room, a familiar cold, clammy sensation grabbed at the crutch and thighs of my theatre greens. I looked down and saw they were soaked in George's blood, an occupational hazard of leaking aneurysm surgery. The changing room furnished me with a shower, but I was forced to bin yet another set of underpants and go commando until reaching home. Once towelled dry and changed into my suit, making sure the trouser zip was firmly closed, I was at last able to sit down and relax with a strong coffee and a fag. Aneurysm surgery always left my nerves jangling from the intense concentration and adrenaline rush; the ten-minute ritual calmed me down and lowered my heart rate. The stress is even worse for a planned elective repair, knowing one false move or lack of attention could kill an otherwise fit and healthy patient. At least with the emergency leaking ones, dying is to be expected and if they survive it's a bonus. A rather sensitive vascular chum once confessed to me that when doing an aneurysm, he died a thousand times. I knew exactly what he meant but made light of it, just to tease him. 'Really?' I said, putting down my pint on the table between us, and frowning with no trace of sympathy. 'I don't … I shit a thousand bricks instead.'

Unusually, it was approaching seven in the evening. My normal post-leaking aneurysm nicotine hit always seemed to be in the dead of night or early morning, with me debating whether to go home for a change of clothes or start the day's work early. I had the weekend off but would check in with ITU before leaving the hospital and check in again on Saturday and Sunday. In between, they knew to contact me if there were any untoward events, like a re-bleed.

George's stars must have been perfectly aligned. He'd made it to A&E, met a registrar who knew what she was doing, had a good crew in place, and the operation had gone surprisingly well. What's more, last time I looked, he was peeing. Always a good sign. George was over the first hurdle. He wasn't yet dead.

The first successful abdominal aneurysm repair was done in 1951, just fifty years before George walked into my clinic. It was a planned procedure, not a rupture, and the surgeon a Frenchman called Charles Dubost. For the graft, he used a length of preserved human aorta from a young woman who had died a few weeks beforehand. Others copied him with variable results, mainly because "homografts" (from the same species) proved to be poor material and much like today, were hard to come by – organ donation after death remains sub-optimal. By the mid-1950s surgeons were routinely using off-the-shelf synthetics and the Dacron graft was born. Rumours abound that in the intervening years, at least one surgeon implanted a graft fashioned by his wife on her sewing machine using an offcut from the tail of his shirt, but I've never found any reputable evidence for this. Once synthetic grafts and the skill to use them were available, vascular and cardiovascular surgery for aneurysms and other conditions, advanced at lightning speed.

Before 1951, various attempts at treating AAAs included simply tying off the aorta, sewing it down to size, injecting the aneurysm sac with yards of fine wire to induce clotting, and wrapping it in cellophane to bolster its strength. The results were universally poor. Albert Einstein had the cellophane wrap, living five years before succumbing to a rupture, though he refused further surgery, maintaining he'd lived his span and preferred to die with dignity.

In 1961, a young American medical student called Tom Fogarty invented the balloon catheter to extricate clots from arteries. Previously, a leg artery for example, blocked by a clot causing impending gangrene, would be cut open along its length for the blockage to be found and removed; a prolonged, hugely invasive procedure with 50:50 odds. Fogarty's catheter could be inserted through a small groin incision, passed beyond the blockage as far as the ankle if necessary, and the balloon inflated and then withdrawn, bringing the clot with it. Simple and highly effective, but no one else thought of it. If you recall, during George's aneurysm repair I was particularly concerned about clots in his leg arteries. Had there been any, Audrey would have passed me a Fogarty catheter to deal with the minor inconvenience.

Fogarty's balloon-on-a-stick idea went on to spawn balloon angioplasty – stretching open a narrowed segment of artery – in all areas of the body. Put a decent sized needle into a convenient artery, often the groin, pass a balloon catheter through it, position the deflated balloon across the troublesome stricture using X-ray imaging, blow it up, and hey presto, the artery's back to normal size. Then, deflate the balloon and withdraw it, job done. The first coronary angioplasty was in 1977, a harbinger of doom for cardiac surgeons whose bread and butter work was coronary artery bypass grafting – split open the breast bone, plumb in a heart-lung perfusion machine, induce a cardiac arrest, then use the patient's own transplanted leg vein to bypass the narrowing in the coronary artery, and hope the heart starts beating again afterwards. A no-contest choice between the two techniques.

Then, someone thought (it's arguable who): howzabout slipping a thin tube made of wire mesh over the deflated balloon? As the balloon inflates to push open the narrowed artery, the wire mesh tube also expands, stays in place once the balloon is withdrawn, and prevents any further narrowing in the future. Would that be a good idea? You bet. The first coronary "stents" as they're called, were inserted in the mid-1980s. Now, it's the norm.

By 1990, someone else came up with the idea of using a larger balloon with a larger wire mesh stent covered in a Dacron tube graft, to fix AAAs. Instead of an open operation like George's, where the Dacron graft is sewn in by hand, the balloon-on-a-stick positions the graft across the aneurysm and is blown up to fix both the graft and wire mesh in place. Called EVAR, Endo-Vascular Aneurysm Repair, the operation is done through two small groin incisions to gain access to the femoral arteries, and negates any need for major open abdominal surgery. It took a few years to catch on because the upstream fishing-hook attachment design wasn't always water (blood) tight, leading to "endo-leaks", further expansion of the aneurysm, and the need for conventional open repair complicated by the previous in-situ endo-graft.

Nowadays, the endo-leak problem has largely been overcome and EVAR for planned AAA repair – and increasingly, emergency leaking ones – has replaced the highly invasive old-fashioned operation. In good hands, it takes about the same time but is far less dangerous, the post-op thirty-day mortality being zero. Hopefully, it has similarly good long-term results. However, because it is such a newly adopted procedure, as Roy would say, *It's Too Soon To Know.*

I do, nevertheless, have at least one reservation regarding the new order. In my last year of practice before retiring, I did perhaps half a dozen elective open AAA repairs in patients who were deemed not suitable for EVAR, mainly because the "top end" of the aneurysm, as viewed on CT or MRI scanning, was too wide or too angled for the technique to be successful. This number contrasts with around twenty a year before EVAR was introduced and even more before the Small Aneurysm Trial publication. My time-expired vascular colleagues would reflect a similar experience. Presently, up-and-coming trainees will be well versed and skilled in endo-vascular intervention, but will be less adept for when, inevitably, an open procedure is required.

George spent several days in ITU, in what the media love to describe as an induced coma. Over a period of many hours, the paralysing drugs and mechanical ventilation were discontinued, allowing him to breathe for himself, even though he was kept asleep with anaesthetic. With his vital signs, fluid balance and urine output monitored, blood clotting and haemoglobin corrected to normal with further transfusions, and countless other tweaks to his physiology, he slowly improved. By the second or third day, the anaesthetic drugs were withdrawn, he woke up, and the endo-tracheal breathing tube was removed. George was going to make it.

Throughout, a rather elegant lady sat vigil at his bedside. Permed silver hair, pearls, twinset, sensible brown shoes, short nails, heavy pleated skirt, minimal make-up, and half-moon gold-wire reading glasses sitting on the tip of her nose – the type of tough, no-nonsense, energetic woman who built the British Empire and won wars. I easily imagined a pair of gundogs sitting obediently at her heel. Clearly from a military background, her bearing and commanding presence terrified the ITU girls. We first met on my Saturday morning visit. Not expecting any relatives at 8 a.m., let alone quasi-Royalty, I was resplendent in an old shirt, jeans and trainers, with a trip to the garden centre on my mind.

She was absorbed in the crossword on her lap. 'Ah,' standing up from the bedside chair, she peered over her glasses to give me the once-over, dropped a neatly folded copy of *The Times* onto her seat, then held out her hand, 'They told me you'd be here early. I'm George's fiancé.' She spoke with a slight Scottish lilt, reminding me of the honeymoon plans, her handshake brisk and businesslike.

'Pleased to meet you, though I wasn't expecting to see you so soon. Have you been here all night?'

'Yes, but no matter. Now, can you tell me how he's doing? He has family abroad and I need to keep them informed. I want to be able to tell them I've spoken with the surgeon.'

'Certainly. Let's commandeer Sister's office and we can have a quiet chat in private,' I indicated the other eleven patients in the unit, the bleeping monitors, the hissing ventilators, the attendant nurses. Commandeer? Had I said that? I was already falling into line.

Sister made tea and then joined us, not as chaperone, but to be kept in the loop. Eileen was easily ruffled if any consultant made promises she couldn't keep. She also knew which cabinet drawer held the tissues. Such meetings tended to be tearful and sometimes hostile, so it was sensible to have an experienced third party. Once sat around the small coffee table, I opened my mouth to begin the introductions.

'Well?' she interrupted, looking directly at me, tea untouched. 'How is he?' her voice now nervous rather than assertive.

'Doing rather well, I think,' glancing at Eileen, who nodded in support. 'Considering the big operation he's had, I'm pleased with his progress, but he's not out of the woods yet.'

'So, I can tell them you said he's doing well? And that you're pleased?' Try as she might, her grey eyes glistened with tears.

Ding! The penny dropped, for me if not for Eileen, who was not entirely in the same loop. This wonderful lady was speaking on behalf of "the family", yet her own heart was breaking. Without any legitimate claim on George, she was left with no other choice; friends, as opposed to relatives, have no legal rights whatsoever. Somehow, she'd blagged her way in. I leaned across the coffee table to hold both her hands in mine. 'Slow down a minute. I know you're supposed to be getting married next week and then go on a coach tour of Scotland. Judging from your accent, I'm guessing that'll be in the Highlands, Inverness or thereabouts, showing George around your old stomping grounds?'

She smiled briefly, making the tears brim over her cheeks. 'A wee bit further north, but you're near enough.'

'George told me everything. So, it's okay to be upset. You must be going through hell.'

'That dear girl ... the registrar ... last night ...' she sobbed with convulsive shudders. 'She assumed I was his wife, and because of her, so did everyone else. I've felt like an imposter all night, but I just can't bear to leave his side.' Then, she pulled her hands from mine, her head went down, and the tears really poured. *The little minx. My bricklayer's mate. She knew the situation. We'd even discussed the inevitable cancellation of George's forthcoming wedding during the quieter moments of the operation. She'd cut straight through all the potential crap and sidelined it. Good for her.*

Eileen, magician-like, produced a fistful of tissues and passed them over. Then, she looked sideways at me, wide-eyed with raised eyebrows. I mouthed, 'Later,' putting a finger to my lips.

It took a few seconds, but then I had it, and spoke to the crown of her head. 'My medical opinion, as George's consultant with full knowledge of his wishes and present circumstances, and because you're due to be married a week from today, is that you should be treated as his wife and partner. That is entirely in his best interests and will aid his recovery. If anyone has a problem with it, I'll deal with them personally.' I looked at Eileen, 'Sister, do you agree?' Finally knowing all the facts, she smiled and spoke loudly, 'I do.'

Once George was woken from his "induced coma", there was some talk of getting the hospital chaplain to perform the ceremony. I told them both it was their decision, but my feeling was since the groom was making such a spectacular recovery, there was no pressing need. In the end, he spent about ten days as an in-patient and they were married a couple of weeks later – about the same time I did the aneurysm patient who took George's place in the diary.

There is one small post-script to tell you. Because they both lived alone and George would need some post-op tender loving care, they overcame their self-inflicted social mores. He was discharged into her custody at her home with explicit instructions not to get mollycoddled to death.

'No lying about in bed or slouching in front of the TV all day, George. You absolutely mustn't be waited on hand and foot, or you'll get clots in your leg veins, and that'll be the end of you. Get out and walk the streets, do some gardening, anything to keep active. You'll get better quicker. In other words, don't allow her to nurse you like a sick puppy.'

As always, she was sitting at his bedside, stately as ever, my advice addressed as much to her as to George. 'Yessir,' he said, taking her hand in his, and giving me a wink. 'But don't forget, it'll be the first time we've been together day and night.'

I suppose here is as good a place as anywhere else to tell you why I adopted vascular surgery as my specialty. In my early years, in common with all junior surgeons, gross haemorrhage – as opposed to minor bleeding – completely, utterly, hand-tremblingly, terrified me. Not a phobia, just lack of experience in how to deal with it and how to stop it, particularly when it was unexpected. You may remember an appendix operation I related previously, when a young woman's belly was unexpectedly full of blood and she ended up scarred for life with a tick shape carved into the skin of her abdomen? Well, she was the catalyst.

That operation had me almost immobilised with fear. The sensation, and the scar I'd inflicted, tormented me for many sleepless nights. How could I set my sights on a career in surgery if bleeding scared me rigid? I resolved to confess my concern to the boss and broached the subject as we were both scrubbing up for one of his lists. His answer was blunt, but incisive as a blade.

'We've all been through the same thing. Make sure you get to do a hands-on cardio-thoracic or vascular job. Preferably both. That'll sort you out. You'll never be frightened of blood again.'

So that's what I did. Not only that, I haunted the vascular lists in whichever hospital I worked. Observing, comprehending, volunteering to assist, learning from master craftsmen, until the fear abated. Bleeding of any sort soon became a minor inconvenience, something to tut-tut about, to sort out and fix. Somewhere along the way, I fell in love with the specialty. If forced to say exactly why, it was the immediacy that had me hooked.

If you remove a segment of intestine and restore continuity by sewing the two ends together, it can be up to a week before the patient's gut starts working again, thereby confirming the operation's been successful. That's why there's an obsessive preoccupation with bowel movements and farting on surgical wards, "Have you passed wind yet, Mr Smith?" Imagine taking your sickly car to a mechanic. He exits the workshop wiping his oily hands on a rag and says to you, 'I've fixed the problem, but I reckon it'll be about next Tuesday before we know if it's worked. As soon as smoke starts coming from the exhaust pipe, you can come and collect it. I'll give you a ring.' That's bowel surgery.

A vascular anastomosis works as soon as the clamps come off, or it should, otherwise you do it again, and again, until it does. No waiting for days. You know it's job done, even before closing the wound. The previously cold white dead leg becomes warm and pink before your eyes, and the pulses return. The graft you've carefully implanted – a segment of vein or an inert tube of Dacron or PTFE (Teflon) – suddenly springs into rhythmic pulsating life, delivering precious blood and oxygen to whichever body part was previously starved of it. Everything about the discipline seemed in my young eyes to be dramatic, exciting, and immediately satisfying. And it was still in its infancy when I joined the club: new techniques; new grafts; novel thinking; good research; lots of ideas to explore. At the time, it dominated the content of all the surgical journals, so when I wasn't doing it, I was reading about it, happily obsessed.

In addition, whereas many of my peers found vascular surgery a difficult demanding mistress and were content to sit back and wait for the exhaust smoke of relatively simplistic bowel surgery, I embraced her, not for kudos, but for the enchanting allure of instant gratification. My butterfly brain, immediately freed from concern for the last patient, could devote itself to the next, and the one after that.

By way of demonstration, I'll finish this chapter with a short tale.

A few weeks before I retired, I helped my registrar do an urgent Fem-Fem cross-over graft. He was a promising lad in his mid-twenties, with good hands and bright prospects. Because he showed such potential, I'd gone out of my way to reduce the list size in order to devote more time and patience to him and the procedure.

The patient was an old man with a blood-deprived (ischaemic) right leg causing pain at rest, a serious pre-gangrenous condition which is both agonising and crippling; he couldn't sleep, let alone walk. The cause of the ischaemia was a furred-up right iliac artery, the one that feeds blood to the leg from the abdominal aorta, where the latter branches into two. The intent of the operation was to steal blood from the good femoral artery in the left groin and feed it to the starved femoral artery on the right, thereby bypassing the blocked iliac – a femoral to femoral, or Fem-Fem graft. In terms of difficulty, for a consultant it was perhaps four out of ten, but for a young registrar, it was supersonic flying.

After an hour, we had both groins open and a graft tunnelled beneath the skin of the lower abdomen, with each end anastomosed to the femoral artery on both sides. On the right side, the last couple of stitches were yet to be inserted.

'Okay, that looks good. Now, you need to briefly release the clamp to check there's good flow and to blow out any clots through the vent you've left open. Make sure–' In his eagerness to please, the lad did exactly as instructed, but a little prematurely. His reward was a satisfying shoosh of high-pressure arterial blood, and a direct hit to the face. 'As

I was just about to say, make sure to hold a hand over it, so you don't get a face full.'

'Sorry Boss.'

'No matter, it's done now. Just lean back, so you don't drip into the wound.'

A nurse wiped a wet towel over his face and eyes, leaving his mask and the front of his blue theatre hat splattered. With a neat steady hand, he inserted the final few stitches before tying the suture with seven throws. Then, he released the clamp and checked his handiwork for leaks and a pulse. 'Seems good,' he said.

'It does.' I agreed. 'But a pulse doesn't mean there's flow, does it?'

'We could use the Doppler, or the electromagnetic flowmeter. That would tell us.' He was suggesting a couple of bits of kit all the youngsters were keen on. Such technology is useful in the correct circumstances, but this wasn't one of them.

I sighed heavily. 'Why not simply look at the feet?' The scrub nurse understood my intention and manoeuvred her tray away from the bottom end of the table. Her runner, a junior nurse, careful to maintain sterility, folded the green drapes back to expose the old man's feet. The left one, belonging to the donor leg, was pink and healthy looking. Good. At least the graft coming from the femoral artery on that side wasn't compromising the blood supply. The right foot was alabaster white and equally as lifeless.

'It hasn't worked,' my apprentice observed with a note of dismay. 'It's still dead.'

'Patience. Have some faith, and watch.'

Everyone in the theatre, from the anaesthetist down to the medical students, peered intently at the dead foot, and in the befitting silence that followed, witnessed a miracle. As the seconds ticked by, the foot slowly suffused with colour. At first, the delicate pink hue of a tea rose was just perceptible, soon to be replaced by a maiden's blush, and finally, after a minute or two, the glowing vermilion of sunrise.

'It's like magic,' the lad whispered to himself, eyes transfixed and sparkling. And in that moment, I knew my mistress had enthralled him too. Beneath the bloodied mask and hat, he was grinning fit to burst.

So was I. Even after thirty-odd years in the game. Absolute, bloody, magic.

9

RESEARCH

We first met at an impromptu booze-up at the Royal College of Surgeons. His name was already familiar. As an undergraduate, along with everyone else, I bought a copy of the recommended surgical textbook, co-authored by him, and like everyone else thought it turgid and unreadable. There's still a copy on my bookshelf for old time's sake.

A tall slim man with a full mop of slightly over-long silver hair, a conservative grey suit, white shirt, and a red tie for a splash of colour, Jack Walters was relaxed into a high chair at one end of the bar, quietly sipping Scotch and casting his gaze over the celebrations. His boyish energetic face and startling electric-blue eyes belied his sixty years. In my memory, he reminds me of an aging hippie turned respectable, but in 1981 – the year Prince Charles married Lady Diana – there were no hippies of his vintage, so he was probably a subversive rebel from way back. Our conversation was short and forgettable – possibly because we were both far from sober – but I thanked him for unwittingly buying me a few beers and told him I needed a research job. He asked me to send him a CV and research proposal.

Over the following few days, I updated the CV and cobbled together a research idea. I won't put you off with the details, but it involved plumbing a heart-lung perfusion machine into legs that had been amputated for untreatable ischaemia. It would make a good experimental model, and suffice to say there is always a regular supply of amputated dead legs. The London Hospital library provided me with Walters' address, and I was astounded to discover he was not only Director of the research unit, but also Dean of the medical school, all this whilst fulfilling his NHS consultant surgeon duties, and no doubt supporting a thriving private practice: if you want something done, choose a busy man. Having sent a covering letter and my bundle of papers off, I got on with the job at The London, continued to scour the adverts, and waited.

If you've ever sifted through a hundred CVs to extract a shortlist to interview, you'll appreciate how tedious it can be. Despite the all-seeing eye of whichever politically correct Big Brother is watching over you – be it racist, sexist, or ageist – you're simply looking for someone who can do the job and fit in. A candidate who ticks all your boxes without the need for expensive advertising and tiresome interviews would be a godsend. Either way, I don't recall an advert, and there was certainly no interview panel, no waiting room filled with other nervous applicants, no personnel lady checking the paperwork. So I never knew if there were any other contenders.

King's College Hospital in Denmark Hill, south London, has an imposing colonnaded facade, much like all the other

London teaching hospitals, though the building itself is a comparative youngster, having opened for business in 1913. The Deanery Office, situated off to the right of the grand main entrance hall, was occupied by a lady with the appearance and charm of everyone's idea of a fairy godmother: white permed hair, an innocent engaging smile, a prim high-buttoned blouse, and a voice like warm honey running over buttered toast. I was to discover her name was Jean and she could, when riled enough to feel the need to protect her beloved boss, snarl and bite like a cornered lioness.

I knocked and put my head around the heavy dark wooden door. Jean was sat behind a desk in the small oak-panelled anteroom, her typewriter stuttering like a semi-automatic weapon set to rapid fire. 'Hello, I'm here to see Mr Walters, have I come to the right place?'

Taking her finger off the trigger, she stood to her full five-foot and waved a welcoming hand at me. 'Indeed, you have. Please come in and take a seat. Can I get you a tea or coffee?'

Pushing the door fully open and stepping onto the deep-pile fitted carpet, I gave her my best smile. 'No thanks, I'm fine. You must be the lady who rang me last week to arrange this visit?' Wearing my only suit, together with the plainest tie, I slid onto one of the five or six upright wooden chairs arranged side by side along the wall opposite her desk. All reminiscent of being summoned to see the headmaster.

'Yes, I am.

'I'm sorry I'm a little early. If it's inconvenient, I'd be happy to push off for ten minutes and come back.' My nerves had me babbling like a moron, and I could have murdered a cigarette.

'No need. Mr Walters is waiting for you. Let me just see if he's ready.' She walked a few paces to her right and pushed open the only other door in the room, 'Your visitor's here. Shall I send him in?'

Jean ushered me into a huge Edwardian-styled boardroom. Long enough to swallow a cricket pitch, a high ceiling with ornate plasterwork and chandeliers, yet more oak panelling, but here lightened by slanting sunlight through tall windows along one side. Large oil portraits of important-looking men lined the walls, but I recognised only one, Joseph Lister, the "father" of antiseptic surgery, who also has the dubious honour of having a mouthwash named after him. The whole decor yelled power and history. Dominating the room, and running almost its full length, was a huge mahogany table with enough matching chairs to accommodate thirty people. Walters was sitting on one of them at the far end, my paperwork in front of him. 'Hello again, thanks for coming,' he patted the leather padding on the chair to his right, 'Have a seat.'

It was a short chat rather than an interview. From the start, he spoke as if the job was mine, telling me at some length about his unit and the different areas of research he oversaw, with an emphasis on Raynaud's. I fleshed out my proposal on dead legs and he listened politely while his eyes glazed over. He insisted all his research fellows should be on the on-call rota, 'It'll keep you in practise and boost your research salary, which is poor. You'd be happy with that?'

'Oh yes. I've been a bit concerned about turning my back on operating for two years or more. I envisaged having to do weekend locum work just to keep my hand in.'

'No need. I've seen to all that. You'll also be expected to attend the surgical unit research meetings, do some teaching, and go to the mortality and morbidity sessions. The last thing I want is for you to lock yourself away in the lab and forget how to operate. Now, I assume you'll be free at the beginning of August. Can you start then?'

'Yes, thank you.'

And that was it. Brief and to the point, with a research job and start date in the bag. At the time, I was stupid enough to suppose it was my glowing CV and magnetic personality that prevailed, together with a huge chunk of luck. But now, years after the event and much wiser, I know it wasn't and never could be that simple. Jack Walters was no fool and wouldn't appoint an underling on the simple evidence of a CV and a natter. No doubt he made direct enquiries at The London and probably elsewhere as to my veracity and worth. The sham interview was designed to back up and confirm what information he'd already gleaned from my former and present chiefs. My CV listed all their names and I'd suggested and primed two of them as referees, who no doubt provided written references. But that would be to nullify the rarefied and cloistered circles consultant surgeons inhabit. They flock together in private hospital operating theatres, surgical meetings, at College and University exams, and most would have crossed paths when they were junior trainees. I've done it; all professionals, and anyone with any sense, does it. He would have phoned a friend.

'Hi, Joe, how's life? Tell me, there's a lad who's applied for a job with me. His CV says he worked for you a few years back. What do you think of him?'

You and Joe go back thirty or forty years, from when you were both at medical school together, or registrars at St. Whoever's hospital and looked after each other's back on a shared rota. You were at his wedding, you're godfather to one of his children, meet him regularly at the private hospital, the College, examinations, socially, and you've trusted him, respected him enough, to ask for an opinion and/or operate on you, your wife, one of your kids, or vice versa. You may also be able seek the judgement of Matt, Marcus, Lucy or Joanna, with whom you have a similar history. Given a sterile, and possibly fabricated CV, what would you do? Yet such activity is widely regarded as a closed shop old-boy network, or elitist. Perhaps in the worlds of merchant banking and politics, it is. But if you're about to take on the responsibility for training a would-be surgeon, who might one day have your life – and, certainly, the life of others – quite literally, in his hands, you want at least a modicum of talent and application to work with. A turd with a perfect CV and good references from people you don't know, is simply a polished turd until proved otherwise. Trainers in any sphere, from bus driver through to nuclear scientist, have a moral and possibly legal gatekeeping responsibility to protect the public from harm, yet some never have the heart or moral fibre to call a halt, to say "enough" to the trainee, and instead shuffle the problem onto someone else. A discreet word with a good mate like "Joe" cuts through any dissemblance.

On the first day, I arrived early and met Walters as he arrived at his morning out-patient clinic. In effect I was reporting for duty and expecting some orders, a plan of action, but it was very understated and typically British. We shook hands briefly. 'I suggest you spend a couple of weeks getting to know the unit and see what takes your fancy. I'll catch up with you after that.' Then, he bustled off to see his first patient.

Dulwich Hospital reminded me of my sojourn at Mile End. A couple of miles from King's and serving as an annex to the main hospital, it was yet another Victorian pile, in itself of some aesthetic worth, but its general appearance betrayed a poorhouse turned infirmary. The Biomedical Engineering Unit was housed in a standalone two-storey building which at one time must have been either an isolation unit for patients with infectious diseases or a nurses' home, both of which performed the same function, though the latter isolated nurses from amorous men. With many rooms of differing sizes, it was admirably suited to host a dozen post-grad engineers alongside their many research jigs and machines. One room, the size of a large kitchen, housed a mainframe computer as big as a delivery truck, floor to ceiling, with just enough space to walk between it and the walls. I was awestruck by its flashing lights and magnificence, but the engineers called it a "stone-age piece of shit" and used tabletop BBC microcomputers instead. Eventually it disappeared, possibly to a museum.

To me, the whole place was a maelstrom of baffling activity with engineering and mathematics at its core. The unit housed its own machine tool shop in the basement, with lathes, huge drills, punches, sheet metal presses, stress testing rigs, and countless other contraptions, all guarded by an old man called Bill who always wore an oil-stained brown lab coat. Bill's job was to protect his precious machine tools from abuse by young engineers, and foolhardy young engineers from the lethal effects of machine tools. An electronics lab with multimeters, oscilloscopes, a dozen soldering irons, cabinets full of chips, circuit boards, transistors, resistors and other wizardry was in constant use. These people were inventing, designing and constructing diagnostic gadgets and instruments prior to testing on themselves and each other: "The diodes in this photoplethysmograph aren't emitting at the right Hertz. Is it a duff batch or the power feed?" A dark room – PowerPoint was yet to be invented – produced slides for presentations at meetings and conferences; that is, if you needed slides, you did the photography and the developing yourself. I felt like an infant transported to an alien planet. My only solace was the other surgeon who was building and trialling a combined carotid artery 3D scanner and flowmeter. An Australian who'd come to England "to cut the poms", he'd already been in the unit eighteen months, with a plan to get his Master of Surgery degree and then go home. Naturally, we ended up in the local pub where he explained the on-call rota and gave me some advice.

'The engineers need us, and we need them. Help them out with patients, clinical know-how, write the medical sections for their papers, and they'll reciprocate. That way we all get our names on the publications. Good, eh? Before you know it, you'll have a dozen papers to add to the CV. Research units live or die on published papers. That's how they attract funding. It's simple maths. More papers equals more research grants.'

I spent a fortnight mooching around, learning names, reading past theses, scientific journals and rearranging pens and pencils on my desk. My desk! I'd never had one before. It was all wood, older than my father, wouldn't have looked out of place on a fly tip, and each of the drawers had its own individual quirky way to yank it open. Abutting a window on the ground floor, it gave me a view of the patchy lawn and weedy flower beds running up to the surgical wing of the main building. By leaning forwards and looking up, I could see a segment of sky with jets approaching Heathrow far to the west. Not only was I effectively unemployed, I couldn't rustle up any interest in my idea of perfusing dead legs – "Sounds a bit smelly for me."

Once a week, the tedium was relieved by seeing real patients for an hour or two in the vascular lab, another in-house room equipped with a treadmill and department-built equipment. They were referred with leg pain on exercise – claudication, from the Latin to limp, and the reason Claudius with his club foot was so named – and needed ankle blood pressures measured to determine the severity and site of furred-up leg arteries, if indeed that was the cause. At the time, a dedicated vascular lab was a novel idea, but now they're widespread.

It was three weeks before I met Walters again. I was heading along a busy corridor toward the hospital canteen for lunch and, by chance, he was walking at his usual brisk pace in the opposite direction. We both came to an emergency halt. 'How's the Raynaud's research coming on?' His voice didn't intone an enquiry. Rather, I had the distinct impression of a command. Or a threat.

'I've read Beamish's thesis and others, spent time swotting up and looking around the unit, and I've a few ideas where to go from here.' Much of what I said was true, though I really didn't embrace the idea of having to do Raynaud's research.

'Good,' he grunted, blue eyes blazing, and strode off. At that precise moment, I decided Raynaud's phenomenon was the be-all and end-all of any young vascular surgeon's existence.

My predecessor in the unit had been collaborating with a young woman called June, an Imperial College engineering graduate who seemed frightfully clever. I say frightfully, because having something of Cheltenham Ladies' College crossed with Joyce Grenfell about her, she used the word a lot, as in, 'Lackers (*that's Lacrosse to you and me*) is a frightfully super game.' Also, whenever she attempted to explain her research to me, I found it scarily incomprehensible. Tall, gawky, and like many impossibly intelligent women, lacking any sense of fashion, she spoke fluent gobbledegook with a corn-popping delivery. I'd already decided whatever she was doing for her PhD was way over my head. Nevertheless, after Walters' veiled threat, it seemed there was no choice other than to get stuck in. June was the only person "doing" Raynaud's and without a qualified clinician to nominally take charge of her volunteer patients, as well as steering her through the medicine and physiology, she'd be dead in the water. Conversely, without her, I'd be sunk without trace. By the time I finished lunch, not only did I understand Walters' ire, I was a man with a plan.

When I found her, June was sitting on a stool in the electronics lab soldering exotic components to a circuit board. She wore a purple hand-knitted cardigan over a cream rose-print dress. The cardigan looked like a reject from a blind-school knitting class for beginners, and the dress just had to be on loan from her mother. Her outfit was accessorized with a green Alice band and a tatty, brown-leather primary-school satchel, slung with a strap from her left shoulder so it rested at her right hip. I held a fistful of paper and a couple of pencils. 'June, what are you doing for the rest of the day?'

She carefully placed the hot soldering iron in its spring-like holder, and with an air of finality, switched it off at the wall socket. Then, with a suspicious frown, turned to face me. 'Nothing now. Why?'

'I'd like to take you to a pub and get you pissed enough

to talk at some simplistic level I can understand.' I waved the A4 sheets as an enticement, 'I'll even take notes.'

Shifting her gaze to the floor, she gave the briefest smile to the lino under her feet. Instinct told me the smile meant she'd been patiently waiting these last few weeks for my epiphany. Or, more likely, she'd grassed on me to Walters and finally knew it had produced the desired result. Then, lifting her head, she refocused on me. 'Super idea. Let's go.'

June proved to have a prodigious appetite for lager, matching me pint for pint, though I preferred proper ale. Over about three hours, I asked dumb questions and she supplied answers a ten-year-old could understand, albeit one with A level physics. Instead of Fast Fourier Transform, she said, "waveform analysis"; for impedance, "damping"; and likewise for a dozen other terms, including gain and entrainment. I wrote copious notes and she added a few diagrams. When it was her turn to quiz me, she plumbed the shallows of my knowledge of physiology and thermoregulation – an endeavour that took about three minutes and offered her no crumbs of comfort. Nevertheless, by the time we'd both drunk too much, it was clear that by working together we could have a fruitful symbiotic relationship, and of greater importance, we thoroughly enjoyed each other's company. At the end of our session, she said, 'For a medic, you seem rather brighter than most.' I reckoned it was the lager talking. The ale in me replied, 'Don't talk bollocks, June. It's just that you've been speaking to me in English for the first time.'

You will have suffered Raynaud's phenomenon in severe cold. Your hands, and often feet, turn white and numb, then, as they warm up, the colour changes to blue and finally red, before settling back to normal. The re-warming phase is often mildly uncomfortable, but overall the whole episode is a short-lived natural response to cooling, far more commonly seen in slim women rather than stocky men. If it occurs frequently – is triggered, for example, by a cool breeze on a warm day or by grabbing a cold spanner from a toolbox – it is, on the face of it, simply an abnormally sensitive response. Yet, it will interfere with day-to-day living: retrieving food from the refrigerator, washing hands under a cold tap, holding a glass of iced lemonade, and as such, is a medical condition. On a more sinister level, it can be a precursor to developing chronic diseases such as lupus, scleroderma and rheumatoid arthritis, or a blood-thickening problem like myeloma or leukaemia. So it has some serious ramifications.

Historically, after all other avenues were explored, patients often ended up in front of a surgeon who would offer a sympathectomy, an operation to cut nerves in the root of the neck that cause constriction of the hand arteries, thereby theoretically preventing any cold-induced spasm. The results were often dramatically good – beautifully warm hands – but invariably short lived (weeks or months) and, nowadays, symptomatic patents are routinely seen by a specialist in rheumatology and offered medical therapy rather than surgery. As far as I'm aware, the underlying mechanism of Raynaud's remains unclear to this day.

June's plan was to measure and analyse human temperature control mechanisms from an engineering perspective. Once I understood the concept, I found it fascinating. A simple painless fingertip probe can give a continuous electronic readout of blood flow traced onto a screen. Since the fingertip is largely skin with a sliver of bone, the trace measures skin blood flow and bops along at about seventy beats a minute, the pulse of the heart beating. But if you watch carefully, the whole trace moves gently up and down about sixteen times each minute; that's breathing causing a decrease or increase in general circulation as blood is alternately sucked into or squeezed out of the lungs. Superimposed onto the fluctuations of pulse and breathing is an even slower one that is harder to spot; about once a minute, the trace moves slowly up and down the screen. Unimaginatively, they're called "slow waves" and are assumed to be thermoregulation, or body temperature control.

Turn on the hot tap in the kitchen or bathroom and you expect it to produce water at around 65C, or whatever temperature you've set the thermostat to achieve. If the hot water in the tank cools down a fraction, the heater will fire up until the set temperature is reached and then turn itself off. Your fridge freezer, central heating and air conditioning function in the same way, the thermostat working as part of a feedback loop, activating or deactivating whatever mechanism warms or cools to keep the set temperature constant.

Those "slow waves" in the blood flow trace are caused by a thermostat in your brain stem turning on and off.

Imagine it, a small collection of temperature-sensitive cells programmed to maintain themselves at a constant 37C and wired by microscopic nerves to the tiny arteries beneath your skin. If the temperature of the cells drops below 37C, they shout 'ON' and all the arteries constrict, preserving and maintaining body heat until their temperature rises to 37C once more. Above 37C, the cells stop shouting and the vessels relax, thereby allowing warm blood to the skin surface where it radiates heat away. All this happens about once every minute, the feedback loop making the mechanism "hunt" around a mean of 37C far more sensitively than any thermostat in your home.

Simple, you may think, and so would I. But engineers like to know if the "shout" is FM (frequency modulated) as in ON….. ON…. ON… ON.. ON. ONONON; shouting more frequently. Or AM (amplitude modulated) as in ON, ON, ON, ON, ON; shouting more loudly. A common misconception regarding home central heating systems is ably demonstrated by my wife. She thinks turning the thermostat dial in the living room to its highest setting makes it "shout" more loudly and urgently to the boiler and will speed the warming process. It doesn't and it won't, respectively, because the thermostat doesn't and won't make the water hotter or the pump bigger and faster; it simply gives the instruction 'ON' for longer, eventually making the living room unbearably warm. At which point, my wife turns the thermostat down to its lowest setting and opens all the windows until she's comfortable, all the while happily oblivious to the concept of feedback loops, and contemptuous of the amplitude and frequency of my objections.

The engineering experiment June outlined was to analyse the blood flow trace in one hand whilst thermally challenging the opposite hand with hot and cold water at different speeds. Get the frequency of the thermal challenge correct, and the rising and falling "slow waves" should get dragged into sequence (entrain) with the alternating hot and cold challenge. And what's more, it worked.

Over two years, we tested normal volunteers; Raynaud's patients; women versus men; pre- and post-menopausal women; complete menstrual cycles on a daily basis; on the Pill and off; with drugs and without; and every permutation we could think of. Patients with Raynaud's and normal women around ovulation displayed significantly abnormal results. Along the way, we published original scientific papers, presented at prestigious conferences at home and abroad, came up with good theories, and generally did a fine job of enhancing the reputation of the unit. No paper was ever presented or sent for peer review without first being given in-house approval by Walters and all the other engineers. Presentations and drafts were usually ripped to pieces and re-edited over and over until they were perfect – length, prose, statistics, scientific method, results and references. An overly busy slide would be derided, as would running over or under time (presentations were strictly ten or fifteen minutes) or fluffing the statistical analysis – all done with humour and generous encouragement.

It was during this period, I met the woman who was to

become my wife. An all-expenses-paid scientific workshop on blood flow physiology and Raynaud's had been organised by an international pharmaceutical company, with around twenty clinicians and pure scientists from Britain and mainland Europe invited to attend. The aim was to present papers, exchange information and foster harmonious cooperation. Held over a long weekend, the venue was the conference room of a plush hotel in the middle of Paris, chosen because it was the most central and easily accessible city for all the delegates. We were put up in the hotel, with lavish dining and entertainment laid on each evening after the hard work was done. She was an attractive physiologist working towards a PhD, and much harmonious cooperation was indeed fostered. What else would you expect in the world's most romantic city? Within eighteen months, we were married.

Six months before the end of the job, I began pulling the elements of my thesis together and writing. Perceived wisdom at the time was that an MS should be 300 pages long with 300 references. It seemed a Herculean task, and one I couldn't tackle during daylight hours because of constant interruptions, tests to do, patients to see, papers to write. My previously bare desk was now castellated with piles of reference books, back issues of journals and other tomes, each with coloured slips of paper marking important passages. A small area to the front and middle allowed space to write or correct another draft paper, or occasionally just to sit and think. The previously clear view of the lawn and surgical wing was gone, but there was still a precious sliver of blue sky.

With no peace to be found during the day, thesis writing took place in the evenings on the dining table at home, the only surface large enough to accommodate the mountain of papers. Armed with a pencil, eraser, a lined notebook and boxed reference cards, I would scribble until midnight, often lubricating the muse with Scotch. Then, the following evening, I stayed on at the unit to use the latest technological advance of its time – the secretary's golf ball self-correcting electric typewriter – and transcribe the previous night's work. It went on for months, alternately scribbling and typing well into the night. On-call weekends were a boon: I could get a serious amount of work done in the deserted unit at the typewriter, while simultaneously dealing with whatever surgical emergencies arose.

Somewhere in the middle of all this, one day Walters found me at my desk. He looked so intent and purposeful that for a moment I briefly wondered what wrong I'd committed. Then, he held out a copy of his co-authored undergraduate textbook to show me the title cover.

'You're familiar with this?'

'Of course. I read it as a student.'

Whereupon he flipped it open to somewhere near the middle, flicked a few pages back and forth until he found the beginning of a chapter, and flamboyantly ripped the book in half.

'It needs revision and the other chap's unavailable.' He handed me the second half, 'You do that lot and I'll do this,' brandishing the first half. 'Nothing fancy, just bring it up to date. Indicate the changes in the text and type the revisions. The publisher will do the rest. Should take about ...' a millisecond passed, 'shall we say six weeks? Then, we'll sit down together, amalgamate both halves and hand it over. Any questions?'

'No, I'm already looking forward to getting started.' And in truth, I was. I mentioned earlier my poor opinion of the book, so in my mind the task was simple. Make it shorter, sweeter, with more headings and more illustrations. The critical question was why he should choose me to do it, though on that point he wasn't forthcoming. But if it meant future students wouldn't have to wade through interminable stodgy text, then I was all for it.

'Good. It won't make you any money. Possibly a few hundred in the first year, but thanks for doing it.' Then, he turned and hurried off at his usual fast pace.

As always with these things, it took longer than expected. The finished product was published a year or so later.

Ten years on, Jack Walters was long dead, but I emulated his ripping-a-textbook-in-half trick to my new co-author and echoed a similar caveat regarding piddling remuneration. 'Don't get your wife all excited. If she starts dreaming of a new set of wheels, tell her they'll be on a skateboard at best.' After eighteen months of self-inflicted torture, a completely new textbook was published. The dedication page says, "To the memory of Jack Walters."

My research post included, as promised, a good deal of emergency and routine surgery, which I was delighted to do. It kept my hand in, and the on-call duty turned out to be a doddle which supplemented the research pay. At that stage in my career, most general surgery fell easily within the scope of my experience, so either doing it myself, or teaching another junior how to do it, was a pleasant distraction from the intensity of research. And compared to the teaching hospital I'd previously vacated, the whole experience was a joy.

King's seemed to be infused with a vibrant energy and a collective wish to be better, more efficient and more learned. Not just better than anywhere else, but an introspective, self-analytically better than they themselves were a year ago, better than they were right there and then. For a start there were no, in my view, mediocre or slow surgeons. The senior consultants were doyens (one was Surgeon to the Queen), the younger ones up-and-coming stars (the Professor was a leading light in breast cancer research). The Liver Unit was first-class, as was liver surgery. Within months of starting my research job, I'd become a regular in theatres, attended the weekly X-ray and surgical meetings, and the monthly M&M (mortality and morbidity) or murder and mayhem session. They were all must-go gatherings for consultants, professors, and juniors of all ranks including students, not because of any edict, but because they were informative, light-hearted, and fun. Sure, there was competitive banter between the chiefs, but that added to the allure, and it was never vindictive. And the overall aim was excellence.

The Wednesday 8 a.m. surgical meetings gave all the many research fellows like me a chance to show their mettle, practise forthcoming presentations to a large audience and field questions from senior surgeons and professors. The X-ray meeting (Monday 7.30 a.m.) was a forum to challenge the radiologists on a recently issued report, ask for an opinion on a weekend X-ray yet to be reviewed, or show one of interest or amusement to the audience. I once took a plain abdominal film of a mentally ill woman who'd swallowed half a dozen ballpoint pens. The senior radiologist, with his usual stern *gravitas*, took several minutes to point out and diagnose arthritis in the hips and spine, calcified lymph nodes (old TB), an enlarged liver (alcohol), fallopian tube clips (sterilisation) and a few other interesting but minor things. His performance had the assembled audience tingling with excitement because the pens were there on the six-foot high projection, clear for all to see, yet seemingly he'd missed them. Finally, he said, '... and of course she's ingested a handful of ballpoints. I assume she was trying to write herself off.'

The M&M meeting was chaired by a senior consultant and was always mobbed. It reviewed all that month's surgical deaths (nearly all expected and inevitable), and any serious surgical complications, (rare, but possibly avoidable with the benefit of hindsight). If the patient was yours, you were expected to explain or defend your actions and say how the situation could have been handled for better or worse. Thus, consultants and lower ranks would speak openly and honestly without fear of censure and everyone learned how to avoid similar traps. In modern "management speak", they were holding priceless multifaceted jewels of unintentional consequences, otherwise known as cock-ups, high into the shining light of publicity and understanding. By doing so, everyone gains. But they were doing it years before it was standard practice, when the norm would be to hide or somehow cover up complications or errors.

About that time, the physicians presented me with a classic Friday evening patient, an elderly man with a bleeding duodenal ulcer (DU) who they'd been treating all week with antacid therapy and blood transfusions. As usual, with the weekend upon them, they handballed him onto the surgeons with a "failed medical treatment" tag, which in other words means, "get on and operate." Physicians absolutely hate handing such patients over to surgeons because it's an explicit admission of their own failure, but they do it readily enough on a Friday evening when it's their weekend off. When they're still on call and attending, they hang on until Monday morning, then take it on the chin and admit defeat, just at the most difficult time to fit a patient onto an emergency list.

I went to see the old boy on the medical ward. He was propped up in bed on multiple pillows, white from anaemia and breathing hard through lack of oxygen to his tissues. His notes told me he suffered from ankylosing spondylitis, a painful arthritic condition where the spinal vertebrae fuse together to produce the classic crooked man, whose backbone is so fixed and curved, his head is level with the handle of the stick he's forced to use. No doubt the bleeding ulcer was at least partly caused by anti-inflammatory arthritis medication.

An ulcer is an open sore, produced when the normal surface covering is eroded by some pathological process; mouth ulcer, leg ulcer, corneal ulcer, cervix ulcer. The duodenum is the first part of the small bowel that accepts food from the stomach, and it's lined by pink intestinal mucosa, similar to the lining of your mouth. A duodenal ulcer in the front or anterior part can erode into the peritoneal cavity and perforate, thereby allowing stomach contents to slosh around the abdomen and produce peritonitis. A posterior ulcer eats into the dense tissue lying behind the duodenum and tends to erode a small artery, which bleeds. The man needed an operation to open the duodenum from the front, locate the posterior bleeding ulcer and oversew it, thereby both closing the ulcer and ligating – strangling – the bleeding artery. Standard everyday stuff.

Later that evening, after he was anaesthetised and placed on the operating table by means of a canvas stretcher, the pillows supporting his head and back were still in place. 'Hang on a minute guys,' I said, 'I can't operate on him like that. Pull out the pillows and lay him flat.'

The orderly and anaesthetist duly obliged, but the patient, or more specifically his fused spine, didn't. He lay there like an acutely curved banana, balanced on his lower back with no means of support, as if stuck in the middle of a sit-up crunch exercise. And I'd walked straight into the trap. There was no way his abdomen could accommodate a standard midline, up-and-down, incision. The space between the lower end of his breastbone and the pubic bone was less than a palm width – nowhere near long enough – so it would have to be a transverse, side-to-side, incision. Not ideal because his ribs and the crest of his hip, or iliac bone, were also vying for space, but once inside I reckoned there'd be enough room for me to do the deed. And anyway, I had no choice but to plough on, otherwise he'd bleed to death. We put the pillows back under his legs and head until he was properly supported in an optimum position. Then, I asked for the knife.

The duodenum is an easy target, laying as it does just beneath the skin and muscle of the upper abdomen, a little to the right of the midline. In this case it seemed about a fathom deep, and with the ribs and iliac bone so close to each other, it was like operating through the slot of a letterbox. The houseman did sterling work with a retractor, accompanied by much sweating from him and swearing from me. As planned, I opened the duodenum from the front to get at the bleed, but the whole duodenum was so ulcerated and fragile it fell apart in my hands. Rather than a disaster, it was a blessing in disguise. The posterior ulcer came into plain view, together with the hissing, pissing bleed. A few carefully placed sutures and it was under control, producing an audible sigh from the anaesthetist, who, up to that point had been struggling to keep up with the blood loss. Then, we all took a short rest, mainly to give the anaesthetist some catch-up blood-transfusion time, and the houseman a break from his arduous toil. Meanwhile, I pondered the situation.

Ordinarily at that point, I'd neatly close the anterior duodenum to restore continuity with the stomach and then close the abdomen. But the macerated bowel was never going to hold a stitch long enough for it to heal, and once it inevitably fell apart again, probably within a day or two, green bile combined with stomach acid would cause peritonitis and kill the patient. So, instead, I completely detached the distended stomach from the duodenum, and from it massaged about a pint of clotted blood into a kidney dish. The now-collapsed and empty stomach was easily plumbed into a loop of the uppermost small bowel. Food would now bypass the duodenum and enter the bowel just a little farther along its normal pathway, yet still be digested normally. This left one remaining problem, the one-inch diameter open tube of duodenum that was already leaking bile and other digestive juices. How to block it off safely?

So long as the duodenal leak is directed to outside the abdomen, the patient is safe, though mildly depleted of fluid and salts, an inconvenience easily corrected with an intravenous drip or oral intake. Atmospheric pressure is lower than intra-abdominal pressure, so if you provide a conduit or drain, fluid will always flow from within the abdomen to the outside world. I used the time-honoured solution of a bladder catheter, a rubber tube that at the pointed end incorporates a water-inflated balloon to act as an anchor and seal. The tube causes an inflammatory reaction in the surrounding tissues, producing an organically constructed corridor of tissue – a fistula (Latin: reed or pipe) – which remains after the tube has its balloon deflated and is removed. The fistula continues to safely discharge onto the skin for a few days and then dries up.

With the balloon of the rubber catheter fitting nicely into the duodenum, and a few industrial stitches to hold it there, the bile was soon draining safely into a catheter bag. The crooked man made a complete recovery, the drain doing its job for two weeks before it was removed without complication. Even so, the case was highlighted at the next M&M session and I needed to defend myself. 'Multiple lessons to be learned,' the chairman intoned gravely. *'Too bloody right mate,'* I thought, sitting down again, relieved at finishing the presentation. Then, he went on to ask the assembled crowd if anyone else had performed surgery on a similar patient, and if so, could they please pass on the wisdom of their experience. A sea of blank faces greeted his request, so he came back to me. 'Is there anything you would have done differently?'

'Swapped my on-call,' produced a ripple of laughter and applause. 'But seriously, if I was faced with another, I'd do a transverse incision without hesitation. It's the only way. Any operation thereafter would be awkward, but possible.'

Throughout the rest of my career I encountered several crooks, and even fewer patients with ankylosing spondylitis, but never again operated on such a crooked man.

To me, Jack Walters was more than a good teacher; he was my foremost mentor, arriving at a time in my life when I needed him most. I could "surge" in the same manner a first officer can "fly" a jet liner, but the problem with inexperience is, you simply don't know what you don't know until it jumps up and slaps you across the face. I was competent and confident, but without the nuances and knowledge necessarily honed from decades of stinging cheeks. The airline captain or consultant's role is to pass on that experience whilst remaining hands-off, but ever-watchful for irredeemable errors. At best, the protégé is unaware of such surveillance or tuition, gets on with the job, inevitably makes some mistakes and learns to sort them out. At worst, he rarely gets a chance to fly, and when he does, is criticised for every move. Walters was very much in the former camp, leaving me to my own devices and only rarely needing to pierce me with his laser-blue eyes when I came close to some disaster or made a gaffe. 'I presume you'll never do that again, will you?'

Of my writing skills: 'No, no, no ... not male and female adults, they're bloody men and women." Or, 'Did you simply throw a fistful of commas at this page, or were they deliberately put in at random?'

By his example, I learned humility, honesty and kindness towards patients and peers, how to teach juniors and students, how to think logically and make decisions. And when necessary, how to be forceful without losing my temper, even though the occasional colourful language has its place. He also showed me a little of how hard he worked.

'This is a list of my private patients and which hospitals they're in.' I'd been called to the Deanery one Friday afternoon in the late summer of my second year. 'I'm away in France for a fortnight from tomorrow. Could you keep an eye on them for me? It's short notice I know, but I've been let down by someone else and you seem ideally placed, living up in Woodford as you do. A few diversions on your way here every morning will get them seen in no time.'

I took the typed list together with the pager it was clipped to. There was a patient in every private London hospital I knew, and one I'd never heard of. 'Yes, of course. I'd be delighted to help.' But then again, how could I refuse? He was my chief, my co-author, and a decent man entrusting me with the shop window of his surgical reputation.

'Good man. And thank you. They're all post-op and very straightforward. You'll be able to discharge them within a week, so it won't be too onerous. That bleep, by the way, is the latest model and it's seriously clever; it shows the phone number of whoever wants you. It's only for private hospital use though, so if it ever goes off, it's one of them calling. Just find a phone, ring the number and you'll get straight through.'

Over that weekend, I made my first daily visits and rehearsed the route, starting near Lord's Cricket Ground in the north, zigzagging through town and finishing opposite the Imperial War Museum, south of the Thames. My sturdy Mini, a third-hand orange-coloured rust bucket, served me well, though was out of place alongside the Jags, Mercs and

Daimlers in the car parks. I wore a suit and polished my shoes – if I was going to screw up, I'd at least look the part. Some of the hospitals resembled brash five-star hotels with Cartier, Rolex and other expensive concessions within the lobby area: they were filled with patients from Saudi and the Middle East. Others were more like private clubs: small, discreet and very select, with the slight scent of old money oozing from the restrained Georgian décor – they housed Brits and Asians. The first trip took the best part of four hours, slowed by the need to read case notes, introduce myself to nurses, and examine the patients. For the most part they were post-op hernias, varicose veins or gallbladders, all of which would now be done as day cases, but back then were inpatients for at least a week. One was an Indian lady who had a partial gastrectomy (stomach removal) for a benign ulcer just a day or two earlier. Not yet drinking or eating, with a nasogastric tube in place and an IV drip to keep her hydrated, I knew she'd be the one to watch. By Sunday, the protracted ward round was down to two hours. My forthcoming weekdays would mean flooring the throttle of the Mini at five in the morning if I was to reach King's before seven.

Monday morning. The sun was up and the traffic sparse so I made good progress, but would the nursing staff and patients expect such an early visit? My concern was unfounded. At the first stop, there were already four or five men in suits wandering around the single rooms, and eavesdropping told me they were surgeons and anaesthetists doing pre-op visits. I recalled the cardiac surgeons at The

London generally did at least one "pump" (coronary bypass) each morning on their way to "proper work," but until then, never realised a very early knife-to-skin time was quite normal in the private sector. Back on the road, every red light confirmed it. Among the stationary traffic, I spied other surgeons and anaesthetists I knew from King's and The London or recognised from surgical conferences. They were everywhere, scurrying around from hospital to hospital, doing a ward round like me or going to a list. And by extrapolation, there must have been many more I didn't spot or recognise. It was truly an eye-opener. Jack Walters and his peers were all on some crazy private treadmill. By possessing the three holy A's – affable, able and available – they attracted private customers like flies and couldn't turn them away. A rumour doing the rounds at that time told of a teaching hospital vascular surgeon who was so bored doing private varicose veins, he tripled his charge as a deterrent – and instantly trebled his workload. Another guy with the same problem gave up the NHS to concentrate exclusively on income-enhancing vein surgery and subsequently named his expensive yacht *Varina*, a tongue-in-cheek salute to the activity that financed it.

As the days passed, the morning excursion shortened as I discharged one patient after another, until, by the start of the second week, only one remained: the post-gastrectomy Indian lady. Her operation was a similar procedure to the crooked man I described earlier. Her stomach remnant was plumbed into the high small bowel and her duodenum was stitched shut, but well over a week since the op, she wasn't progressing as expected. The nasogastric tube still produced volumes of green fluid, and if it was left in place but closed shut with a spigot, a prelude to removing it, she vomited similar amounts. Clearly, the stomach wasn't emptying properly – not uncommon in the first few days due to swelling at the anastomosis – but this had lasted far too long. An intravenous drip maintained her hydration and the blood tests were good, but I harboured nagging doubts regarding her nutrition. If she didn't pick up soon, she'd need intravenous feeding. I was also considering a barium meal X-ray to see where the blockage was – loops of small gut can twist – and wondering about the legitimacy of me, a junior surgeon, doing a re-operation in a private hospital. Discreet "what if" enquiries back at King's told me it was impossible. It must be a consultant.

A long chat with the senior sister in charge, a woman with decades of experience, resulted in a plan of action. 'The problem is the woman's a bit precious and won't shift herself. She lies in bed all day like a dead duck, refusing to get up and walk around. I've told her, moaned at her, dragged her into the bedside chair – everything I can think of – but she puts herself back into bed. She needs to move.'

Post-op is not a time to lay about in bed. "Up and at it" is good for the lungs, the heart, the gut, and just about everything else, yet some patients don't win prizes in the up-and-at-it stakes, preferring instead a dying swan routine. 'Okay, I'll read her the riot act. In the meantime, can you get hold of some really stodgy porridge?'

Sister smiled in recognition of an old trick I'd learned

from some equally old surgeons – it gives the stomach something to get its teeth into, so to speak – and porridge was what they all used to stimulate propulsive contractions, open up the anastomosis and get things moving. 'Our chefs can provide anything and everything. It will be here as soon as you've gone.'

So, I read the riot act to the Indian lady, threatening further surgery and all sorts of horrors if she didn't take her drip stand for a walk ten times a day. Sister provided five-star restaurant quality porridge, stripped the bed bare each morning and forced her into the shower each evening. It worked. By the Friday, she was ready to go home, but for some domestic reason elected to go the following day. She was happy, I was happy, Sister was happy. But the following Monday morning, fresh back to work from his holiday, Jack Walters was exceedingly unhappy.

It was yet another summons to the Deanery from his secretary, Jean. When I arrived, she didn't know the reason for the call, 'But …' she gave me a sly grin, 'as you would say, you're in deep shit for something.' I'd already guessed as much myself.

Sat behind his desk at the far end of the boardroom, my entrance produced an instant tirade. 'They told me that woman didn't go home till Saturday. There was no reason to keep her in that long. What the bloody hell were you playing at?' He must have been making some phone calls. Either that, or he was already back on the early morning private hospital tour.

Walking the length of the room, I halted in front of the

desk, not bothering to sit. If I was in for a carpeting, I'd take it on my feet. 'She developed efferent loop obstruction with everything coming up the NG tube and nothing going through. It's all documented on the fluid balance charts and in the notes. It went on for a week or so, but she got going after the Sister and I, if you'll forgive the expression, kicked her arse into gear. I managed it as I would for any other patient. All the rest were no problem.' Fishing out a sheet of paper and his pager from my pocket, I placed both on the desk. 'This is your list of patients with my written comments beside each. My intention was to catch up with you later today and run through them all, but you've rather beaten me to it.'

He calmed down a smidgeon. 'I've never seen an efferent loop obstruction in one of my patients before. Are you certain?'

'Last Monday, I was on the point of ordering a barium meal.' I shrugged my shoulders in a conciliatory "shit happens to the best of us" gesture. He simply harrumphed and indicated I could go.

A couple of weeks later, he handed me a rather generous cheque, 'That's for looking after my patients when I was on holiday. It will show in my accounts as an assistant fee, so it's up to you if you want to tell the taxman.'

'That's kind of you, but I wasn't expecting any payment. And it's far too much.'

'No, it's not. And don't bloody argue, just take it. By the way, that gastrectomy woman is doing well. She asked me to say hello and pass on her thanks to you for bullying her.'

10

NEARLY THERE

With the first draft of the thesis almost written and the research post coming to a close, I needed to find yet another job to complete my surgical training.

It would have to be a senior registrar, one rung beneath consultant level. The alternative was a lecturer post, the academic equivalent, but with an onus on further research and teaching. My previous experience of academic surgery elsewhere was far from good, but the widespread pursuit of excellence at King's had pushed me beyond that prejudice to the point where I now embraced it. Not only that, a lecturer job became vacant at King's just when I needed it. It was pure happenstance, but the whole situation was perfect for me. I knew the job, the hospital, the chiefs, and by staying put wouldn't have to sever my ties to the guys in the research unit. June, my lager-drinking buddy and research partner, still needed some support and continuity. She was a year off finishing her PhD and could best do it without having to induct another rookie idiot like me.

The outcome of my application to the British Medical Journal advert and full panel interview was, I suspect, a shoo-in. Better the devil you know who's good enough, rather than the one you don't, who might well be outstanding on paper and at interview, but forever remains an unknown wild card. On the day, I recognised all the other suited and booted applicants sitting in the waiting room. Many were members of the "perforated condom" club or Slome-Stansfield graduates, others I knew from various vascular and surgical conferences. We greeted each other and chatted amicably, wishing 'Good luck,' and asking, 'How'd it go?' as each departed for a twenty-minute scrutiny and then returned to wait for the panel's decision. Looking around at my fellow candidates, I remember thinking they were all good enough to do the job. Yet there was I, the guy on the inside track, the bookies' favourite, known throughout the hospital for better or worse, and as such, the only runner with absolutely everything to lose. If I didn't get appointed, the shock waves within the tiny world of surgery would tarnish me forever. I'd be the man King's rejected after two years virtually in post. For the other rejected candidates, it would be a case of "Better luck next time." For me, it would be total annihilation. "If King's let him go, why would we want him? He must be seriously flawed." My paranoia proved unfounded, and when invited back to see the panel it was smiles and handshakes all round: 'We'd like to offer you the position. Do you accept?' You betcha.

In total there were five of us, two lecturers and three senior registrars, all in pristine white coats with nothing but a pen in the breast pocket and an expensive stethoscope in the waist. The clinical roles, like the dress code – with obligatory club tie and cufflinks – were indistinguishable, with each individual navigating his final four years of training. The rotation comprised three in-house firms, plus one in Brighton on the south coast or one at The Brook in southeast London. So, in any one year, three of us would be at King's and the other two out in the sticks. The lecturers spent a year in the professorial unit doing breast and vascular, whereas the SRs weren't duty bound, particularly if their interests strayed beyond those subjects. But in practice, they were keen to bag a couple of internationally known professors for their CV, so happily obliged. In any case, all the different disciplines came under the umbrella of General Surgery and we were expected to be better than competent in all of them. The only exception was liver surgery, which specialised in transplants, complications of cirrhosis and excision of liver tumours, but nevertheless was included as part of the rotation, if one was so inclined.

The surgery was all standard everyday stuff, but the real surprise was how little we saw of whichever King's boss we were working for. That's not an accusation of absenteeism on their part, but a reflection of how busy they were with other responsibilities, and how much trust they put in us. For example, I worked for the vascular Professor for a year, but only ever saw him in theatres on two or three occasions. I did all the other operating and most of the clinics. My fellow SRs reported a similar experience during their tenure with him, yet at the time he was pioneering and promoting deep vein thrombosis (DVT) prevention with a missionary fervour which took over most of his life, as well as a great deal of time and effort within the surgical unit conducting numerous clinical trials. If you've had an operation in the last thirty years, you'll recall the white stockings and heparin injections to stop potentially lethal leg vein clots. You can thank my former chief for that. His efforts have by now prevented millions of post-op deaths worldwide.

Mind you, the three of us at King's were happy to be left to our own devices. It meant lots of operating, lots of responsibility, and little interference. We were like three musketeers, self-supporting, watching each other's back, consulting together on how different bosses liked things done, and generally running the show. A joke doing the rounds back then concerned a consultant surgeon who was approached by NASA to undertake a perilous journey to the moon and perform an emergency appendicectomy.

'My fee will be ten thousand pounds, up front, with a five pound tip.'

'Sir, that seems a reasonable price for risking your life to help us out,' the American answered, '... but why the five pound tip?'

'If he makes it back, that's what I'll give my senior registrar for going to do it.'

In retrospect, I'm sure we were deluded to think that as senior registrars we were acting autonomously. During my own consultant years, I left many competent juniors to do lists and clinics without me. It induces confidence and provides experience, but it's hard work picking appropriate lists and then pacing the theatre corridor getting prearranged clandestine reports from your regular anaesthetist-cum-spy on how the tyro is performing. 'She's doing okay, so piss off. Anything untoward and I'll call you.' Or, 'I think you'd better get in here, something's bleeding.' Clinics were less immediately angina-provoking but required careful and time-consuming reviews of notes made and decisions taken, together with the occasional alert from my secretary who audio-typed letters to the GP. 'This is odd. He's done something you don't normally do.'

The plain and simple medico-legal fact is that consultants are responsible for everything done by junior doctors or other agents in their name, so unless you have a penchant for regular court appearances, it pays to be vigilant. A junior doctor, if you need reminding, is any doctor who isn't a consultant, whereas "other agents" pretty much includes anyone else who performs a service at your behest. An example of the latter would be the scrub nurse who counts the swabs and instruments at the start and finish of every procedure to ensure nothing has been left behind. He or she then informs the surgeon, 'All counts correct,' and the appropriate box on the post-op form is ticked. However, in one place I worked, the SR had cause to ring his highly respected boss one evening, and I'm not making this up.

'Hello Sir, sorry to disturb you at home, but I've admitted a fifty-year-old woman with intestinal obstruction following a gallbladder removal done two years ago at this hospital.'

'And?' *Meaning, why are you bothering me with such a simple matter?*

'Ah ... well ... the thing is, the X-ray clearly shows a Roberts forceps within the abdomen.' *A type of stainless-steel clamp, about a foot long.*

'Oh, Christ. Which idiot left that in?'

'Er ... you did, Sir.'

'Shit.'

Any medic would immediately blame the errant scrub nurse, but the patient, the family, the public, the press and the law, blame the surgeon, because he is responsible and he'll be the one in the dock. In practice, such cases are usually settled out of court for large sums because they're legally indefensible, but the ignominy hangs over the surgeon like a dark pall forever. Similarly, there are tales of juniors amputating the wrong leg, removing a fallopian tube instead of the appendix, or doing perfectly good operations on the wrong patients, the list of screw-ups being as endless as it is varied. So, to cut a long diatribe short, only a fool gives his juniors autonomy. The trick is, like the airline captain, to allow the first officer to believe he's doing all the work but be ready to grab the controls at a moment's notice. You probably remember the name Sully Sullenberger, the airline pilot who found himself in charge of an Airbus A320 glider in January 2009. But can you recall the name of his equally praiseworthy first officer? No, you probably can't, because Sully was the captain, the one responsible for his plane, crew and passengers. Yet if he hadn't made the correct decision and pulled off that spectacular ditching, if everyone on board and hundreds more on the ground had died at a crowded New York city crash site, you'd be even less likely to remember the first officer's name, because Sully would be a world-famous pariah. It's a fine line between respect and contempt, and the chief always shoulders the blame along with the credit.

As Walters' SR, each week I did my own list, he did a teaching list with the registrar, and all three of us operated together on Friday afternoons for something big, like an aneurysm. Though with the pressures on him from the Deanery, he would often start things off and then disappear for some important meeting or other. After a while, he simply told me to get on with it.

'I've organised an extra list next Wednesday afternoon,' he cornered me at the end of a morning clinic. 'It's a renal patient and a bit unusual, so I could do with your help if you're free.'

Walters had never asked me or anyone else for help. If the registrar or houseman weren't available, he would co-opt one of the ever-present medical students to assist, or happily proceed with the scrub nurse. Typical of the many old-school surgeons back then, he'd done a stint in the armed forces and trained at a time when anaesthesia was at best hit-and-miss, so accurate speedy surgery became a necessary virtue. As a result, he was lightning-fast and extraordinarily skilled at doing pretty much anything on his own. Most assistants simply leaned on a retractor, but if they understood what they were witnessing, saw a supreme

master at work. So, whatever he was up to, if he w
me to be his wingman, I reckoned it was wa
"unusual". And it couldn't possibly be my surgical prowess
he was after, so it had to be my intellect, my contemporary
knowledge, or simple moral support. 'I'll have to rearrange
a few things, but I'll make it,' I said, adding that I knew
nothing of any renal referral, and shouldn't I be the one
organising extra lists?

'It's a patient in the private wing, so I have all that under
control. All you need to do is turn up. He's a young man
with right renal artery stenosis and refractory hypertension.
Balloon angioplasty didn't work so he needs an open
reconstruction. But something's not quite right about the
whole thing.'

The patient in question had a narrowing (stenosis) in
the artery to his right kidney, as shown on an X-ray with
radio-opaque dye injected. This situation will reduce the
blood flow and pressure to the kidney, fooling it into
believing the blood pressure throughout the whole body has
fallen. The kidney "knows" it can't work without a good
filtration pressure, so spits out hormones which raise the
blood pressure (hypertension) until the kidney is content
with its own supply, thank you very much, but meanwhile
the heart is working overtime and the brain is in danger of
blowing a gasket and stroking out. I suppose you could say
kidneys are selfish sods in that regard. The physicians tried
reducing the blood pressure with medication, but it didn't
work (refractory, from the Latin for stubborn), and in
collusion with the radiologists, failed to balloon the

narrowed renal artery back to its normal diameter. The surgical plan would be to sew a Dacron patch into the artery and thereby correct the narrowing. All of which is a common enough scenario in a sixty-year-old smoker with hardening of the arteries, but in a seventeen-year-old lad? No way. As Walters said, something didn't smell right. What's more, it was a nightmare of a private patient: complex, failed therapy, far too many unknowns, with surgery being the last resort. Private practice is supposed to be straightforward and easy, not walking blindfold into a minefield of possibilities. Clearly, my presence was requested for moral support.

At the appointed hour, the lad was anaesthetised and positioned for surgery left side down with the operating table "cracked" in the middle in an inverted V shape, thereby stretching his right flank wider than it would be when simply lying horizontal. The incision through the skin and underlying muscles stopped short of the peritoneum, the sac of flimsy tissue enclosing the gut. By simply pushing the peritoneum forwards the whole retro-peritoneal area opens up, allowing a reasonably generous amount of space in which to operate. With the patient being young and slim there was little retro-peritoneal fat, what butchers call suet, so within minutes of starting the procedure Walters was carefully holding the kidney in his hand and making rapid progress toward the renal artery and vein, situated deep within the wound. That's when it all went pear-shaped.

'WHATEVER YOU'RE DOING, PLEASE STOP

NOW.' The yell was so loud it echoed off the tiled walls, making the point of origin unclear. Even so, Walters' hands froze, and slowly, gently, he withdrew from the incision. The consultant anaesthetist, one of the regular vascular crew and usually completely unflappable, put his head over the green top-end drape. 'Sorry Jack, whatever you were doing just then put his blood pressure through the roof. Can you leave off a few minutes while I give him a cocktail of drugs to get it lower? And if it's any help, the last time I saw something like this, it turned out to be a Carcinoid tumour. Bloody physicians ...' Shaking his head, he slipped from view.

Carcinoid tumours are often diagnosed from the anaesthetist's behaviour. They're rare, but normally arise in the gut, often presenting with intestinal obstruction or appendicitis. As the surgeon manipulates the tumour during removal, vaso-active chemicals such as serotonin get pushed into the bloodstream in mega quantities, causing arteries throughout the body to constrict and the patient's blood pressure to shoot up. The anaesthetist then panics, bobs up and down and screams "Stop!" Such a reaction is so reliable it's completely diagnostic, immediately forming the thought bubble "Carcinoid" in the surgeon's mind. Walters caught my eye and the glance between us confirmed our mutual second thought. This wouldn't be Carcinoid. Not here in the kidney.

Five minutes later, we were given the go-ahead and went for it, at a snail's pace. Lightly, delicately, Walters isolated the blue renal vein and circled it with a nylon tape sling to hold it to one side, better to get at the artery. But the artery wasn't there. In its place was a gold-yellow walnut-sized lump. He prodded the tumour with a fingertip and produced the desired result, a disembodied voice from the top end, 'The pressure's up again, whatever you're doing.'

'It's adrenal tissue,' Walters said, unnecessarily. 'Must be an adrenal rest.'

The golden colour gave the game away.

The embryological development at the back of the abdomen, what will become the retroperitoneum, is a bit of a nightmare to comprehend. Suffice to say the kidneys and gonads (ovaries or testicles) develop into recognisable organs from simple streaks of genito-urinary cells running alongside the spine. As the embryo grows, the kidneys appear as if by magic and generally are situated where they should be, but it's not uncommon to find a kidney in the pelvis, or the two kidneys joined into one large horseshoe shape, and many other variations on the theme. Similarly, the ovaries and testicles form beside the spine, and then migrate south, though testicles have a much longer journey and sometimes fall short of their final destination: undescended testicles ("Doc, 'is balls 'aven't dropped.") provide much work for paediatric surgeons. Somewhere in this potpourri of primitive cells, the adrenal glands develop and eventually adorn the top of each kidney like a yellow tricorne hat. By the way, ad-renal is ad-kidney in English, as in ad-jacent, near to. Anatomists simply have no imagination.

Adrenal glands, along with cortisone and other

important chemicals, produce a substance you will know, having often experienced its effects. It's the fight or flight hormone that kicks in when danger threatens – heart-thumping, pulse-racing, sweat-running, white-looking, hands-shaking, mouth-drying, pressure-raising, panic-inducing, body-trembling … adrenaline. Somewhere during the lad's embryological development, a few cells destined to become adrenal gland wrapped themselves around his right renal artery, thereby producing an anatomical remnant (or rest) that grew and constricted the vessel.

No wonder the previous attempted balloon angioplasty didn't work. No balloon could ever shift the nubbin of yellow tissue surrounding the artery. And the physicians must have experienced a hairy moment or two, judging by the anaesthetist's response to the gentle fingertip prod. When the balloon was placed in the renal artery by the radiologist, he was attempting to dilate a narrowing in much the same way furred-up coronary arteries in the heart are treated. But the renal artery itself wasn't diseased. The real problem was the tumour surrounding and squeezing it so tightly, though neither the radiologist nor the physicians knew this, because on the X-ray all they could see was dye outlining a seemingly narrowed artery. It must have been all-round adrenaline overdose time when the balloon distended and compressed the aberrant adrenal tissue. The lad's blood pressure and pulse would have skyrocketed, along with all the other adrenaline-induced symptoms. Likewise, the physicians, seeing the dramatic reaction the balloon produced in their patient, would have feared for his life and panicked with a similar response. The balloon, as they say, would have really gone up.

My thoughts were probably echoing Walters', but the problem remained. Like defusing a bomb, it needed handling with care or the explosion of adrenaline into the bloodstream could blow the lad's brains out. After some discussion, the anaesthetist injected a whole load of beta-blockers and anything else he could think of to counter the adrenaline rush. Then, Walters took a small "mosquito" forceps and insinuated it between the renal artery and the lump, establishing a plane of cleavage before cutting through the "doughnut" ring. It sprang apart to reveal a normal healthy artery pulsating within. A few more deft cuts and the whole doughnut was released and removed. It took several minutes, but by the time it was finished, I could swear the gasman had chewed his fingernails down to the knuckles.

A short time later, he'd stopped chewing and was feverishly infusing fluids in a fight to bring the now dangerously low blood pressure back up to normal. The operation had clearly been successful, yet I'd been no more than an onlooker throughout.

As if on cue Walters said, 'Do you mind finishing this off for me? I've a meeting to get to.'

Afterwards, I hung around the recovery room until the patient woke up. He was okay, no stroke and compos mentis, so I wrote the op notes, filled out the path forms and made a mental note to include the private wing on ward rounds for the next week.

Early spring, 1985: Bruce Springsteen was topping the album charts with *Born in the U.S.A.*, the BBC TV soap opera, *EastEnders*, had just aired for the first time, and the date for my thesis viva/interrogation was set.

Two vascular surgery professors from London teaching hospitals would perform the task. I knew both by repute, as well as seeing them in action at various clinical and scientific conferences. One would instigate "The UK Small Aneurysm Trial" which forever changed the timing of treatment. The other was widely respected for his surgical flair and intellect, and was a leading light in carotid artery surgery. Medical students and junior doctors called him "Smiling Death", a nickname bestowed because of his elegant manner and sardonic rictus when examining for the University and College of Surgeons. I'd heard many a failed candidate moan, 'Smiling Death did for me.'

Our paths had crossed before at a prestigious Surgical Research Society meeting. The SRS was *the* place for professors and other luminaries to present their latest work, all done through the mouthpiece of juniors who presented the papers. In reality, it was a bear pit, where research fellows like me were sacrificed for the amusement of our elders, who fought petty disputes or bloody warfare though the medium of disparaging comments and criticisms aimed at their proxy. It was a fascinating testosterone-fuelled spectator sport – unless you were the bear – and much good science was aired. I'd just finished a ten-minute perfectly timed, well-rehearsed and flawlessly given presentation to the Vascular section and stood centre stage at the podium, my final slide still shining on the huge screen behind me. Then, the lights went up in readiness for five minutes of usually hostile questions. No problem. I'd been fully prepared back at the research unit and understood the statistical methods like a pro. Out of a hundred or more in the audience, Smiling Death stood up from his seat. The chairman of the session pointed to him, 'Professor, you have a question for the speaker?'

'Thank you, Mr Chairman, though it's more of an observation than a question.'

'Please, carry on.'

'Well, I don't know about anyone else …' the Prof theatrically panned his gaze across the assembly, simultaneously waving an all-encompassing arm, then he turned to me and smiled, 'but I for one haven't understood a word of what's been said for the last ten minutes.'

Blind panic and the sound of my jaw bouncing off shoelaces make any personal recollection of what came next rather hazy, but the account I give here is supported by reports and comments received from fellow sacrificial bears at the post-mortem in the bar that evening. I spotted a whiteboard with pens at one side of the stage, the sort of thing normally used for messages to the audience: "Will Mr Bloggs please contact his secretary. Urgent". Thankfully, it was clean. Then, the long chats I'd had with my co-researcher June came to mind, along with her easy-enough-for-a-moron-to-understand diagrams and graphs. At the time, I thought it divine inspiration, but it could equally have been Satan's work.

Out of my mouth came something like, 'Yes, I appreciate it can be difficult to grasp the concept of this inherently basic analysis of blood-flow waveforms, but if the chairman would kindly allow me to quickly use the whiteboard, I'm sure I can simplify it for you.'

I glanced at the chairman sitting comfortably at stage right. He seemed to be smirking, though I didn't understand why. He nodded, probably unable to speak, so I made my way to the whiteboard and reportedly gave Smiling Death a four-minute primary school lesson, complete with June's drawings and graphs. When it finished, the chairman rescued me by announcing there was no time for further questions and thanked me for the presentation. No doubt, he led the polite light applause as was normal etiquette, but all I remember is slinking away from the stage like an escaping snake, low, quick and slithery. Now, two years later, I was about to get my comeuppance for unknowingly upstaging one of my examiners.

It was a Friday afternoon in the Professor's office, not far below the top floor of St Thomas' Hospital; two seats on one side of a low coffee table with me opposite. I'd spent weeks going through the thesis to the point where I could quote most of it word for word, and then done the same with all the references, photocopies of which were in the bulging briefcase at my left ankle. It didn't feel like an examination. Two hours or more drinking tea and chatting amicably with my interrogators as they went through the opus line by line, asking for clarification on different points, me, defending the use of one reference over another – all very cosy, learned and gentlemanly. Then, the knife came out with the inevitable smile. He reached into his own bag and produced a small slim book that I recognised as an Academic Press production with the catchy title of *Non-invasive Physiological Measurement*. The topic was of such narrow interest, having read it I doubted if the print run was more than a few hundred, probably enough for one copy in every big physiology institute worldwide, with a few leftovers for family and friends. Not a best-seller then, yet here was the only other copy I'd ever seen.

'You've read this book I assume? You cite it in the references.'

'Yes, of course I've read it.'

He passed it over. 'Show me where you claim it says your method measures flow rather than fluctuations in volume.'

It took me about five seconds to find the relevant passage. I shoved the open book back to him across the coffee table, 'There it is, the two concluding paragraphs on the left-hand page, but the meat is in the main text.' *He's trying to make me out to be a liar.*

'Thank you, I have also read it. But the author says, "It is logical to assume ..."'

'Well it is, for all the excellent reasons and experimental data he mentions. That's why I cited him. And all his research is published elsewhere in peer-reviewed journals ...'

We railed at each other for twenty minutes, with him repeatedly arguing against "assumptions" and me fighting an increasingly desperate urge to wipe the smirk off his face with back of my hand. I think I finished with something like, 'Well, the best man on the planet thinks it's logical, his peer reviewers think it's logical, everyone in the field thinks it's logical, and I think it's logical. Frankly, Sir, I don't know why you can't agree, and I can think of nothing else to say to change your mind.'

At that point, the other Professor, who'd been a complete bystander in the rumpus, jumped in like a man determined to separate two fighting dogs, though he spoke directly to me. 'I think that particular aspect has been thoroughly discussed, and we've been at it now for ...' he checked his watch, 'well over two hours. I think it would be good idea if we all have a break. So, if you don't mind, perhaps if you take a walk, freshen up, that sort of thing, and come back in say, fifteen minutes? Just knock on the door and walk back in. Okay?'

I found a window with a spectacularly elevated view overlooking the Thames. Various boats, up and downstream, ploughed serene aqueous arrowheads, each one silver-sparkling in reflected sunlight. Westminster Bridge, and on the other side of the river, Parliament Square, were clogged with week-end traffic and teeming pedestrians, all scurrying to the siren call of Poets' day – piss off early, tomorrow's Saturday. A couple of cigarettes later, the seething fury in me lessened from blistering red to cautionary amber.

'We both think your thesis is a significant and novel

contribution to the literature,' the dog-fight referee said, after we resumed. I sensed the "but" coming, 'But ...' *smarmy sod, this is his doing,* 'we also agree some form of clarification regarding the volume versus flow issue is needed, so ...' *Why can't you just grow some cojones, you wimp?*

I butted in, ignoring the monkey, and spoke directly to the organ grinder. 'What would satisfy you?'

In short, the argument was: if method A correlates with B, and B correlates with C, it's logical to assume A correlates with C. Smiling Death wanted the assumption removed with some experimental demonstration that A showed a direct and highly significant correlation to C. Over the weekend, I calmed down – a lot – and concluded it was a valid request, which also made good science. Not only that, if the matter wasn't resolved, June would most likely get a similar drubbing when her PhD was examined.

Within a few weeks, with me fitting things in alongside my full-time clinical job, we'd designed and tested our experiment on each other, everyone else in the research unit, a few patients and several visitors – particularly if they were women – to make up the numbers. The correlation between method A and C was, as expected, nigh on perfect – so good, in fact, I believe June wrote it up as a paper and sent it off to her favourite engineering journal. Meanwhile, rather than simply add an addendum to the thesis, I knocked out a completely new draft to include the correlation experiment – not a quick fix, even with an electric golf-ball typewriter – made three or four copies and took the whole lot back to the binders. Then, I resubmitted it with a covering letter addressed to both professors.

A few weeks later, the man himself rang me at work to say everything was now acceptable and congratulated me on a job well done. In turn, I graciously offered my heartfelt thanks for his ultimately correct guidance and wisdom. The thesis was undoubtedly stronger as a result.

When my MS certificate arrived the whole research unit, in keeping with long-held tradition, held a monumental piss-up on me at a cheap local Italian restaurant. Jack Walters brought his wife, got pleasantly sozzled, said a lot of nice things about how wonderfully we all worked together, and even chipped in for some of the booze bill.

Lecturer duties were mainly confined to teaching medical students, organising the weekly department meetings, and being dogsbody for the clinical part of the finals exams.

Late spring each year, volunteer surgical patients were needed to fill a vacated ward for the duration of the exam. To prevent any possibility of cheating, the patients had to differ from morning to afternoon session, and from day to day, so large numbers were required. The medical school provided appropriate clerical assistance to run the show, but patients were the cast members and without them there could be no performance. Consequently, the Lecturer's role was to browbeat the medical staff into recruiting scores of suitable volunteers from clinics, waiting lists and the wards.

Furthermore, because the examiners would be professors and consultants from other teaching hospitals, the quality of the clinical cases and smooth running of the exam was a matter of some kudos for the surgical unit. After all, if you're opening the shop to scrutiny from outsiders, the display cabinets need to be in good order and show the brightest trinkets. For example, a post-op liver transplant complete with appropriate scars would trump an ingrowing toenail.

Once the clinical cases were recruited, the exam itself was a simple caretaking job. Ensure unlimited access to tea and biscuits for the examiners, provide them with a good lunch, be present to sort out any problems, and look after the patients, each accommodated in a curtained-off bed. Strolling up and down the ward and eavesdropping on proceedings behind each curtain allowed some timely interventions. More than once, I needed to reassure a terrified patient their simple fatty lump was quite benign and the medical student's diagnosis of rampant cancer wildly incorrect.

One volunteer patient was a young man in his late teens with a silicone testicular prosthesis. He'd previously suffered a twisted testicle (*sadly, not the name of a heavy metal band, though it should be*), a condition where the testicle rotates around its attachment to the spermatic cord, strangles the blood supply, turns gangrenous and needs removal. Common practice is to insert the silicone cosmetic device to "balance things up". Of itself, it's a simple smooth ovoid of the correct size, but devoid of any other anatomical features such as spermatic cord or epididymis. I thought him extremely brave – or innocent and uninformed – to volunteer to have his private parts assaulted by a succession of nervous examinees. His curious anatomy really shouldn't have presented any problems for final year students, especially the men, but many were flummoxed, and the two examiners became increasingly irritated by inane responses to their questions. Enter the next candidate, a guileless young woman who seemed to have dressed for Sunday school. The exchange as heard from my side of the curtain went like this:

Examiner 1: 'Please examine this gentleman's testes and comment on your findings.'

Candidate, following a long pause while conducting the examination: 'Well ... after a thorough inspection and palpation ... and judging from experience ... I don't think the left testicle is entirely normal.'

Examiner 2, in a despairing tone: 'How much experience have you had?'

Candidate: 'None, I'm afraid.'

Towards the end of my time on the King's rotation, I began to feel disenchanted with London. Apart from a couple of years in the suburbs of Sussex, the whole of my adult life had been spent in the sprawling city. The metropolitan existence had once captivated the naïve eighteen-year-old student, but after fifteen years and approaching my mid-thirties ... well, familiarity brings 20/20 vision. Crowded with mostly brutish people, paralysed by stagnant traffic, no definable seasons except dirty dusty hot or miserable cold dark damp, it was expensive, noisy, tiresome, tiring, dangerous, lawless, and oppressive.

King's College Hospital is situated on the edge of Brixton, then a poor borough with a large African-Caribbean community and high levels of unemployment, endemic theft and violent crime. The police were regarded as racists specifically targeting young black men, and coupled with real or perceived social injustice, the whole simmering area ignited in the riots of 1981 and 1985. Brixton became known locally as "The Front Line" and by default King's was the casualty clearing station for the war zone, though Tommy's hospital to the west also took some of the fallout.

Cannabis was so freely available that even the middle-aged West Indian cleaning ladies working within the hospital regularly brought in ganja chocolate brownies to eat during tea breaks, which probably accounted for their charmingly languid attitude to life and work. Famously, one of them disrupted the Professor's rounds with her mop, clanging galvanised bucket and gentle rendition of Bob Marley's *No Woman, No Cry*.

Standing fully erect at about five foot eight, he puffed up his chest, stuck out his jaw and accosted her, 'Madam, would you please desist. I am the Professor of Surgery and I'm trying to do a ward round.'

She was what you'd call a big Mamma, and at just over six foot and two hundred pounds, it was never going to be a fair contest. She gave him a long slow look up and down, but mainly down, as if considering that very same question, while at the same time weighing up the consequences of physical, rather than verbal abuse. Happily, she took the verbal option, adopting a defiant stance with one large fist wrapped around the mop handle, the other wagging a chubby index finger at his nose. 'Misser, Ah dun't care if you'ze de Lord God Ormighty hisself. Ah gotta get dis floor clean, so you'ze jus' betta git outa ma face an' leev-mee-be.'

Out on the streets though, drugs and gang culture produced a regular stream of knife and firearm injuries to Casualty. Sporadic skirmishes between rival gang members who accompanied their fallen comrades prompted the presence of burly security guards within the department itself. It was an edgy place to work, particularly on dark evenings when most of the trouble arrived. Medics and nurses kept an eye on each other and rushed to help when needed. One night, I saw a drunk/junkie/mad guy give a nurse a backhander to her face as she was showing him to a cubicle. Within milliseconds of her scream, he was on the floor beneath a scrum of white coats, each one giving payback with interest before throwing him out through the door. Such assaults on staff were common, yet all this violence happened against a background of dealing with normal everyday emergencies.

Standard surgical protocol was to explore all penetrating injuries, a time-consuming and often fruitless exercise if the knife or projectile was shown to have caused no deep injury to vital organs or vessels. One senior registrar was coerced or offered to go on a short fact-finding trip to the Groote

Schuur Hospital in Cape Town, infamous for dealing with dozens of such patients every day. His report, with appropriate photos, delivered at a Wednesday morning surgical meeting, was revolutionary. At the Groote Schuur, unless a patient was clearly bleeding out with some catastrophic internal injury, all casualties were sat in a row and simply observed. If they "wobbled on their perch" or looked likely to fall off it, a closer examination was warranted, and appropriate treatment given. Belly wounds received no treatment unless they developed peritonitis or signs of bleeding. Wounds to the chest had a drain inserted for a pneumothorax (punctured lung) or fluid shadow (bleeding) as seen on an X-ray and returned to their seat for further observation. The photos showed a line of at least twenty chairs along one side of a long corridor, mostly occupied with young black men. 'This ...' the SR declared, 'is the observation ward.'

His recommendation was to adopt the South African approach at King's and the statistics backed him up. We all readily accepted, though it was easier to provide trolleys rather than chairs. The number of exploratory operations for malicious penetrating trauma dropped significantly, though my feelings of futility at having to do such surgery in a "civilized" society never wavered. Man's seemingly limitless capacity to inflict senseless brutality always fills me with a forlorn hopelessness wherever I see it, either on news bulletins or at my fingertips.

One patient, a white man in his early twenties, was admitted after being assaulted in a pub car park by a gang. He'd taken a severe beating, been stabbed and slashed repeatedly, and finally someone "kneecapped" him from close range with a shotgun. All the injuries were peripheral – none to the chest or abdomen – so were theoretically survivable, an indication, I was told, of a controlled punishment attack rather than attempted murder. Nevertheless, he lost a lot of blood and the scalp lacerations and shotgun wound were still bleeding. A deep stab wound to one buttock was also hissing scarlet, no doubt from the superior gluteal artery.

As the Casualty team inserted lines and began infusions of blood and fluids, I stood back and pondered my options. He had to go to theatre of course, but on my own it would take about three hours to patch him up, and while I was sorting out his bum, the scalp and kneecapping wounds would still be bleeding. Another pair of educated hands would speed things along and save needless blood loss. Ding! A quick phone call to the doctors' mess secured the services of the ENT senior reg, 'Yeah, okay. I've nothing better to do and there's bugger all on telly worth watching.' And so, at around midnight, three SRs (don't forget the anaesthetist) began throwing a couple of hours of their life away, using thirty years of collective experience to salvage a pitiful wretch who'd been found guilty of some underworld crime and viciously punished by a gang of lawless hoodlums. And tomorrow, and the day after that, it would be some other poor sod with similar injuries but a different story. The relentless inevitability of it was, and no doubt still is, soul-destroying.

The patient was face down on the table, a position that

gave me access to his buttock while my ENT partner worked on the deep scalp wounds. 'These have been done with a Stanley knife,' he opined, 'I can feel the gouge marks in the skull bones.' Meanwhile, I extended the buttock wound with a scalpel and came to the same conclusion. My incision was as neat and sharp as the original wound. Once I'd found and secured the gluteal artery, I closed the skin and we rolled the patient onto his back. Work now started on the leg, with the ENT man assisting.

The shooter missed the kneecap. I suppose in the general ruckus, with the victim wearing jeans on a dark night, it wasn't easy to hit the mark, even from close up. Just above the kneecap the skin and flesh were gone, as if a small shark had taken a bite and retreated with a mouthful of thigh. I'd been worried the femoral vessels and sciatic nerve would be shredded, but the tough young bone of the femur protected them. Much of the blast had in any case gone to the lateral side where no important structures lay. It was what John Wayne would call "a flesh wound", but a bloody big one, the size of my fist. The hole was cleaned of dead meat and foreign material (scraps of denim, lead shot, cartridge wadding) and left open to heal naturally. Another forty minutes suturing the numerous other wounds and we were finished. By three, I was back in Casualty seeing a normal emergency, the anaesthetist was doing another case, and the ENT man was in bed.

The following morning, the patient was on a ward with an armed policeman sitting guard at his bedside in case the assailants reappeared. It wasn't an unusual sight, and these days it's even more frequent. The patient looked like shit but would survive. Knowing detectives would inevitably be all over the case, I kept the cartridge wads and some lead shot in a plastic specimen tube, and sticky-taped it to the op notes. I also told the houseman to ask the hospital photographer for forensic-quality pictures of every square inch of his body, with close-ups of all wounds. Coupled with good quality notes, I reasoned the plods should have all the evidence we could provide, and specifically, no need to bother me. And they didn't for a year or more. By which time I was a consultant …

Tuesday, ten o'clock at night, and a loud urgent banging on the front door. There was a working bell and a knocker, but no, whoever it was preferred a solid fist on wood. Perhaps there was a fire, a neighbour in trouble; what else could it be? Rushing to the door, I flung it open. A big copper was standing on the doorstep, blinking in the light from the hall. What crime had I committed? Which relative was dead?

'Good evening, Sir, this is for you,' he handed me a large brown envelope with my name and address printed on it.

'What's this?'

'It's a summons requiring your presence at the Old Bailey at eight o'clock tomorrow morning.'

'That's ridiculous. I can't be there at such short notice.' *A morning list was scheduled with no one else to do it.*

'If you don't appear, you'll be in contempt of court. Then, we'll have to arrest you and escort you there. Do you understand?'

'Well … yes. But what if …'

'My job's done then, Sir. You have the summons and understand the consequences. Good night to you.'

With no idea what it could be about, the contents of the envelope failed to enlighten me. Regina v somebody I'd never heard of – at least it wasn't me – together with instructions to turn up and how to get there. With no choice, a few phone calls later I'd cancelled the list and the rest of Wednesday.

I was outside the appropriate courtroom by eight and on my own, the impressive hallway deserted in my vicinity. So, I loitered, assuming whoever wanted me would find me. Nothing. A peek into the courtroom confirmed it was empty. Should I wait inside or out? I decided on out. Various barristers in wig and gown hustled past, but no one stopped. By nine, a few shady-looking characters were hanging out with me, each appearing similarly lost, and none looking remotely legal. Being the only person in a suit and tie, I recalled an old joke which made me smile (I'm a Scouser by birth): What do you call a Liverpudlian in a suit? The accused. Perhaps that's why they were all avoiding eye contact. Another half hour passed. By now, I'd attracted enough for a football team, plus a few reserves, but they were a motley bunch.

A flustered barrister finally arrived. Short, slim and about fifty, with a huge bundle of notes under his left arm, he was whispering my name to anyone in the squad who would listen. I lifted a finger and he joined me, leaning against the cold marble wall. 'Thanks for coming,' he shook my hand like a dog wags its tail, pleased to see me. 'You're on at ten. Have you prepared?'

I was going to ruin his day, payback for ruining mine. Beyond incandescent and approaching meltdown, I related my visit from the police with as much malice as hushed tones could convey, '... So, no, I'm not prepared, and I have no fucking idea why I'm here under threat of legal action.'

Perhaps all barristers play poker, or a poker face is part of the job. His expression remained blank; no sympathy, no shock, zip all. 'We still have a few minutes. Come with me and I'll get you a coffee.' I expected a private room lined with legal tomes. He led me to a filthy public area with a grubby lino floor, plastic furniture and a slot machine dispenser. He paid. After clearing away the previous occupants' debris, we took an empty table. 'I could reschedule you for tomorrow if you like.'

'What I'd *like*, is to know why I'm here. And *fuck* tomorrow. I'm not putting up with this farce two days running. I cancelled an operating list and a clinic to be here today. I'm not doing it again for tomorrow.' My outburst made no obvious impression on him. The poker face seemed painted on.

'You operated on Joseph Bernard Loggs, also known as Bernie.' It sounded like an accusation.

'No idea. I've operated on lots of people.'

'It was an assault.'

'A lot of them as well. Look, let's save some time, shall we?' I tapped the pile of paper laying on the table between us, 'I assume somewhere in there is an operation note. Let's see it.'

It took a lot of shuffling for him to find it. While

waiting, I sipped the watery coffee and concluded his poker face wasn't an affectation, but the product of an empty mind. 'Ah, here it is,' he said, rotating the bundle and pushing it toward me.

My notes were clear and comprehensive, with appropriate diagrams. It was the kneecapping lad. The date was over a year past, but I remembered all the details. 'You should also have a bunch of photos and samples of wadding and lead shot?'

'Yes, the pictures are in there, together with a ballistics report.' For a fleeting moment, he sounded almost enthusiastic.

'So why do you need me?'

Deflated again, he checked his watch, 'Can we talk on the way? Time's pressing.'

In the space of a two-minute walk I learned three things. He was prosecuting for attempted murder (acting for the Crown; pay peanuts, get monkeys). I would add "colour" and expertise to his case. And the summons arrived late because, apparently, I was a hard man to find. Since I was already trapped I didn't bother to challenge him on this, but reasoned if the police could track me down just twelve hours earlier, they could have done it twelve days, or twelve weeks ago. Even without the extended powers of the law, a call to the GMC would easily suffice, or a look at the electoral roll. And as a last resort, the taxman never fails.

In the witness box I swore the oath and gave my name, rank and credentials. The judge was either very shrewd or already appraised of my legal kidnap, 'You don't appear to have any medical notes to refer to.'

'No Sir (*or should that be M'lud? Damn, too late now*), I was given short notice to be here and consequently had no time to get hold of a copy.'

His grey bushy eyebrows raised a little. 'When *were* you requested to appear?'

'I had a summons served on me by a policeman at ten o'clock yesterday evening.'

The eyebrows took a nosedive to meet the reading glasses perched there, and he rounded on "my" barrister to give him an enormous bollocking of legalese. It was a masterclass in genteel finesse. Without raising his voice an iota, or allowing any ire to surface, he questioned the barrister's behaviour, training, character, lineage, mother's profession ... and generally called him an arse in all but name. I suspect it was a bit of theatre for the benefit of the defence lawyers who must have been put on the back foot by my sudden appearance, but completely shared the sentiment. Then, he turned and gave me a benign smile. 'Given the circumstances and your lack of preparation, do you, nevertheless, still feel able to aid the court?'

'Yes Sir, I've seen my operation notes, recall the case clearly, and I understand everything is documented in the bundle (*my own legalese was coming on leaps and bounds*) should I need to refresh my memory.'

'Thank you.' Then, he blew the whistle and the match kicked off.

It was schoolboy league level and a waste of my time. "My" guy described Loggs' injuries at length, and asked me if they were individually or collectively lethal. I replied that without treatment, possibly. The other side asked if they were survivable with no treatment and received the same response. I told them both I acted as well as any other competent surgeon, and with foresight furnished comprehensive notes, photographs and physical evidence to satisfy the inevitable legal enquiries. Questions regarding my role as a surgeon and the evidence I submitted were fair game. Anything beyond that was the remit of a forensic expert. But it didn't stop them asking. No, I do not know how far blood splatters from a shotgun wound. No, I do not know how long it takes to bleed to death from a femoral artery wound. No, I could not hazard an educated guess. Eventually, the questions dried up and I was dismissed. The kneecapping lad had stolen another four hours of my life.

But far worse, and what riled me most, was my attendance at court caused half a dozen children to have their operations postponed for no good reason.

My increasingly jaundiced view of London life was also influenced by having my first decent second-hand car, a Ford Capri, stolen from the hospital car park. The police contacted me a fortnight later to say they'd found it. 'Great, where and when can I pick it up?' I asked, assuming it would be in a car pound somewhere. 'We don't have it. It's a burnt-out wreck on a Brixton housing estate.'

I also had my wallet stolen, twice. The first time from

the locked on-call room – he came in through the window – and the second time from my stolen car where I'd left it in the glove box for safekeeping. As ever, it wasn't the lost cash but the missing bank cards that caused the most grief. Oh yes, I almost forgot, my replacement car lasted a week before a side window was smashed and the radio nabbed. And my short litany of sorrow was being inflicted so frequently on countless other people, it became a shoulder-shrugging part of normal life. The price paid for living in the big city was to be a victim of crime, no more remarkable than seeing a black cab or a red bus in the street. On the brighter side, at least I wasn't mugged at knife point or blown up by the IRA, which in the early 80s was doing its best to make London a no-go zone. The bombs in Oxford Street, Hyde Park, Regent's Park and Harrods caused many tragic deaths and injuries, but everyday life was also frequently disrupted by suspect devices and false alarms.

When Jack Walters announced his approaching retirement, several seniors and other colleagues tipped me the wink to be his successor. I imagine they saw me as the dream candidate for my dream job. I still had a strong allegiance to the research unit and, with Walters gone, it would need an equally enthusiastic lead clinician to take his place. Also, I'd pretty much become his clone regarding my way of working, thinking, and operating; not a bad role model to emulate. But the thought of spending the rest of my life at King's and in the environs of Brixton filled me with dread. By then, I also had my wife and a baby daughter to add to the reckoning, and simply couldn't condemn them to the same fate. A child needs green fields, fresh air and sunshine to thrive, not grime and crime. I needed out of London altogether.

11

BELLYACHE

I t was a domiciliary visit requested by a worried GP. The patient lived on the edge of town and couldn't drive. Would I do a home visit after work? Such trips were relatively common, particularly to nursing homes or housebound elderly folk. It was quicker and easier for the consultant to travel than arrange transport in the opposite direction. By their very nature, home visits were often to socially deprived areas, so it made good sense to have locking wheel nuts and an alarm system on your car.

On this occasion, it was a pleasant surprise to find a modern terraced house in a well-heeled area, with a Mini parked on the driveway. A concerned and heavily pregnant young woman answered the door with an effusive welcome. Wearing a flowery Laura Ashley smock dress, and with bare feet, she led me through the hall to a modest neat living room. In his late twenties, the husband was sitting on the edge of the sofa, clutching his belly, doubled over in pain, and gently rocking like a metronome. I stood in the doorway and quietly observed. After a minute or so, his pain subsided and he was able to sit upright. 'Thanks for coming. I'm sorry to drag you out here but as I told the GP, I couldn't safely drive to the hospital in this state, and my wife can't fit behind the wheel.' At least the mystery of the car sitting on the driveway was solved.

Slim and fit, he looked more anxious than unwell, and although three days' worth of stubble blurred his chin, he was scrubbed clean in fresh jeans and a tee shirt. Smooth hands with clean manicured nails betrayed an office job. 'Well, let's start by all three of us sitting down and having a chat. Then I'll examine you.' He worked as a junior accountant for a big local firm. The wife was a primary school teacher. He'd had bellyache for two weeks and been off work because of it for one. It was getting worse. 'Describe it for me.'

'Like someone grabbing my guts and twisting them.' As he spoke, he made a fist with his right hand, screwing it into his midriff. 'It lasts a minute or two, then relaxes, then comes back again. Could it be phantom labour pains? I've heard some men get them in sympathy with their wife.'

I ignored the first-child lunacy. 'What about food? Any relationship to eating?'

He looked sheepish. 'If I stick to tea and soup, the pain's bearable. But I was so hungry this morning, I had a bacon sandwich for breakfast and since then it's been really bad. It's coming back now, actually. Excuse me, I need to get up and move around.' He strode about the room, grunting gently to himself with discomfort, before doubling up and sitting down again next to his wife, who was near to tears. Another minute and it had passed.

'Are you scared to eat?'

'Yeah, but I have to try. I've lost half a stone since it started.'

'Any vomiting?'

'Not so far.'

After asking him to take off his tee shirt and lower his jeans, I laid him flat on the sofa and knelt on the carpet to do an examination. The skin around his umbilicus showed irregular brown-red pigmentation, which I recognised as erythema ab igne (Latin: redness due to heat). Other than that, there was nothing abnormal to see or feel. No distension. No lumps or bumps. No hernia. Testicles normal. No enlarged glands in his neck or groins. No anaemia. I had a stethoscope with me, usually more of a calling-card credential than a useful tool, but now I pulled it from my suit pocket and used it. The gurgling bowel sounds were loud and overly active.

'It's been going on longer than two weeks, hasn't it?' I pointed to the pigmentation on his belly, 'The hot water bottle you use to ease the pain takes longer than that to turn the skin brown.'

His eyes widened at the depth of my perception. 'Okay ... I'll admit it. It's been about a month, but it wasn't so bad at first. I was hoping it would just get better.' Then, ignoring me, he sat up and reached to his wife, sitting in the armchair I'd recently vacated. She was quietly sobbing. 'I'm so sorry darling,' he said, holding her hand and stroking her large bump. 'But I couldn't burden the two of you with my troubles, could I? You've enough to contend with.'

The sweetheart interlude gave me the opportunity for some serious logistic thinking. It was clear the couple were in the first throws of love, marriage and soon-to-be parenthood, but she was facing the possibility of being widowed forty years too soon.

He was a tough cookie. A constricting midgut lesion was progressively narrowing to produce worsening colic, and the hyperactive bowel sounds told me his gut was working harder than usual to push food through the tight segment. He was hungry but scared to eat, knowing it would eventually produce intolerable pain, always a Ding! red-light sign, as is the brown pigmentation. Hugging a burning-hot water bottle to counteract even worse pain from elsewhere is a metaphorical emergency call for help. No anaemia, so given his age probably not cancer, though there were a few rare ones to consider. Crohn's disease was a possibility, but this was rapid onset with no prolonged history. I could fart around arranging a barium meal X-ray, it might show the where, but not the why, and he'd still need surgery to diagnose and remove the problem …

Now, leave me planning what to do with our man, and consider a splinter in your finger.

Not only do you sense which finger it's in, you also sense, perhaps to a millimetre or less, which part of your finger it's irritating. Furthermore, from experience, the nature of the pricking discomfort tells you if it's a tiny sliver of wood or a metal shard. You're able to say to anyone who cares to listen, a doctor perhaps, "I have a splinter in my left ring finger, just to one side of the nail. It's so sharp it feels as if it could be metal." Indeed, we can pinpoint to a greater or lesser degree of accuracy, the site and nature of a stimulus anywhere on the skin. Without any knowledge of anatomy, we can conclude all our skin, including the mouth and anus, must be teeming with sensory nerves relaying highly accurate information to the brain. And we'd be correct. It is.

So far so good, but you'll never hear anyone say, 'I have pain in my appendix,' or, 'I can feel a stone rolling around inside my gallbladder.' Why is that? After all, we do feel pain in our belly. If, like me, when young and foolish, you've ever had six pints of ale followed by a vindaloo on a Friday night, you'll recognise the insidious onset of upper abdominal pain which warns of the imminent need to talk to God down the big white telephone. If however, you managed to keep such an evil concoction on board overnight, lower abdominal gripes the following morning acted as an urgent call to stool and could be severe enough to leave tooth marks on the toilet door handle. On a slightly dissimilar note, women feel period pain in the lower abdomen, and when men get a blow to the testicles, the intense and weirdly sickening pain is felt in the back and mid-abdomen. Obviously, our gut and other internal organs must have some nerve connections to the brain, but they're nowhere near as good or as site-specific as the skin. That's because the nerve supply to the gut is very primitive, having its origins in the likes of worms and sea cucumbers, which are little more than a length of gut with a mouth at one end and an anus at the other.

Mind you, would you want a nerve supply to your

insides that is as sensitive as that to the skin? The answer, on reflection, is probably not. Apart from it being a waste of brain space, is there a need to feel food travelling inch by inch through the bowel, or know when your gallbladder contracts? Clearly not. If everything is working tickety-boo, why use up valuable grey matter recording the fact? This primitive nervous system autonomously controls all the stuff we're not usually consciously aware of, such as gut motility, blood pressure and temperature. So, if you don't have much, or any consciousness to start with, such as a worm or sea cucumber, an autonomic system makes perfect sense. No, that's an oxymoron ... an autonomic system is the natural solution, no sense or consciousness needed. And, lo and behold, we've inherited one from a sea cucumber. Isn't evolution a wondrous thing?

Your idea of guts is multiple loops and coils of intestine, all pink, shiny-wet and slithery, yet it's all one single straight tube, one gut with no plural "s". Different parts of the tube are modified for different functions, so it doesn't look the same throughout – the stomach doesn't look like the small bowel, which doesn't look like the colon. But from an evolutionary and embryological perspective, it's a single tube made up of three parts: a front bit, a middle bit, and a back bit; or foregut, midgut and hindgut. Each segment has a single main artery and vein with a single primitive visceral nerve running alongside – plumbing and electric wiring in the same conduit. The nerve and blood vessels branch repeatedly like a tree, but all the branches arise from a single main trunk. And that's it. All coiled up and crammed into the abdomen, the gut appears complex but it's actually quite simple.

The three nerves don't generally talk to the brain but when they do, the only thing they can say is, "PAIN!" But it's *all* the foregut, or *all* the midgut, or *all* the hindgut that's talking. It's like getting a phone call to tell you there's a pain *somewhere* in Scotland, end of message. That's not to say it's always severe pain, mild discomfort in your belly is common. That second helping of pudding has a way of letting you know you've eaten too much, or the out-of-date soft cheese from yesterday has given you the squits today, and don't you regret it.

The brain identifies the call as visceral pain felt in the upper, middle or lower abdomen, corresponding respectively to fore, mid or hindgut. Put the palm of your hand on your upper belly just below where the breastbone (sternum) ends; that's where you get fore-gut pain from the stomach, duodenum, or gall bladder. Slide the palm down so it's now over your belly button; that's the site of midgut pain from all the small bowel and a good length of colon. Palm down further still to just above the pubic bone, and you're on hind-gut territory; the left colon, rectum, bladder and uterus. So, the site of visceral pain can tell your doctor, and you, which segment of gut is sending out a Mayday call. It's not overly specific but at least it differentiates Scotland say, from England or Wales, and we can't confuse the need to vomit with the urge to take a dump or have a pee.

The nature of the pain is also made simple by the fact it

can only be two types: continuous or intermittent. Continuous implies inflammation such as appendicitis, or prolonged ischaemia (lack of blood). Intermittent is what we call colic, waves of griping pain caused by excessive contraction of the bowel as it pushes food along or tries to overcome an obstruction. We all experience colic occasionally – too many plums, green apples, a dodgy curry, gastroenteritis or diarrhoea. It's basically cramps of the gut muscle due to it working too hard, like calf cramp caused by excessive exercise.

So, there you have it. Our loved-up friend told me his pain was midgut colic made worse by eating solid food. I surmised a worsening constriction somewhere between the top of his small bowel and his left colon. The next bacon sarnie could be the one to block his gut completely. He needed a look-see laparotomy. Whatever the underlying cause, I'd deal with it once I opened his belly.

After sharing my conclusions with the couple, I used their home phone to call the hospital and speak to my houseman. 'He'll report direct to the ward. Admit him, nil by mouth with a drip, and add him to tomorrow afternoon's list for a laparotomy. Theatres will probably go apeshit at the size of the list, but tell them to take it up with me in the morning. If they argue, say you're just following orders and it's not your problem. Oh yes, one more thing, let the on-call registrar know you've admitted him. If he deteriorates overnight, I want to know about it.'

The transport issue was solved by his parents-in-law

who lived nearby. Mum would come to live with her daughter; Dad would be the taxi driver. Yes, I did wonder why the solution wasn't forthcoming prior to my visit, but at least I didn't need to add chauffeur to my to-do list.

In the event, it turned out to be a Meckel's diverticulum (after Johann Meckel, a German anatomist, 1781–1833). Unless you're a medic or biologist of some description, you've probably never heard of it. It's a remnant of the embryonic vitello-intestinal duct, which again is also completely meaningless, until I tell you that vitellus is Latin for yolk, as in egg yolk. Just because your mother didn't lay an egg like a hen and sit on you for nine months, it's easy to forget you still developed from one, and it had a yolk to provide nourishment to the embryonic you. The yolk was connected to your intestine by a duct which usually disappears long before birth, but two percent of us have a two-inch souvenir attached to the small bowel about two-foot north of the appendix – known in the trade as the rule of two's. This short cul-de-sac (diverticulum), about the size of your thumb, is generally a trouble-free curiosity, but in our man the Meckel's contained some acid-producing cells which caused an ulcer together with scarring and a stricture. It was an easy task to cut out the diseased segment of bowel and sew the two ends together. His gripes were cured immediately, but it took a few days before he produced any exhaust fumes and solid food was back on the menu.

Yes, you were once connected to an egg yolk, which might come as a shock. I also compared your mother to a hen, which may offend you and your nestlings, but embryology lays bare the links to our common primordial ancestors in a strangely disquieting way. So, to add further insult to injury, you should also know that during the period you were plugged into an egg yolk, in common with all vertebrates, you also had the gill slits of a shark and a short puppy-like tail.

The developmental path from fertilized ovum, to embryo, to healthy baby is both rocky and complex. It takes a lot of cell division to grow from a pinhead to a baby in nine months, and each time a cell divides DNA transcription errors can happen. Half of spontaneous abortions (miscarriages) in the first trimester have chromosomal abnormalities in the "products of conception", a term used because the embryo has decayed beyond, or is too small for anatomical inspection, so only cellular DNA can tell the tale. But that's only in women who are known to be pregnant and report a miscarriage. Far more unreported late or delayed menstrual bleeds undoubtedly add to that number. Even so, many babies with non-lethal embryonic abnormalities survive to full-term and can be treated with surgery. Some are relatively common such as harelip and cleft palate, but most, like residual gill slits, are quite rare. And we all retain a memento of our puppy tail. It's that pointy bone you can feel in your bum-crack which we call the coccyx (Greek: *Kokkux*), because it supposedly resembles a cuckoo's bill.

I once saw a woman in her mid-thirties who'd been referred to my clinic with faecal incontinence by her GP.

Shy and retiring, she was unmarried, short on social skills, and still lived with her parents in a farmhouse, deep in rural Sussex. Her overpowering mother – the farmer's wife – accompanied her. During the preamble she informed me her daughter had suffered lifelong incontinence, but it was only now problematic because a boyfriend and potential suitor was on the scene. I guessed the daughter, a child of the early 1960s, was probably a product of generations of rural inbreeding.

On examination, with a nurse chaperone, I expected to insert my gloved and lubricated right index finger into her anus, but there wasn't one. Not even a dimple in the skin where it should have been. Further probing revealed her rectum was connected to the back wall of her vagina. To be blunt, she crapped through her vagina, and had done since birth. Without an anus, there was no other route for faeces to exit.

Such an arrangement is the norm in most vertebrates (birds, amphibians, reptiles), where the common excretory and genital cavity is called a cloaca (from Latin for sewer). Mammals – vertebrates which secrete milk – are a fortunate evolutionary exception to this rule, for which I imagine, you will be eternally grateful. There are though, some strange primitive misfits like the platypus and spiny anteater (Greek: *monotremes*, one hole), that not only have a cloaca, but also lay eggs and sweat milk onto their belly from where their youngsters lap it up. And therein is a clue to the evolution of normal mammalian breasts: they are highly modified sweat glands. Strange to think human breasts, the focus of such intense social and sexual interest, are merely sweat glands.

But to return to the point, human embryos have a cloaca, and a persistent cloaca is a rare developmental anomaly that is obvious at birth (no anus) and surgically correctable. Why it had taken thirty-odd years for the family to seek treatment wasn't forthcoming, but I reasoned it was probably a home birth without a midwife, and what happens in the farmhouse stays in the farmhouse. I sent her to St Mark's Hospital, then in City Road, London, an historic postgraduate institute for diseases of the colon, rectum and anus, and where Charles Dickens was both a patient and patron. After much consultation, it was decided to leave her be. Even after surgical correction, a considerable undertaking, with no functioning sphincter she would remain incontinent and no better off.

With a shrug, Mum took her back home, never to be seen again.

The suffix "–itis", means inflammation. Some are in common usage – dermatitis, conjunctivitis, arthritis – and others less so – balanitis, blepharitis, myelitis. The term was coined by ancient physicians to describe the response of living tissue to injury or infection. We all have personal everyday experience of the inflammatory response, be it from an infected spot, sunburn or a sprained ankle. It's heat, redness, pain and swelling, or if you're a citizen of early

Rome, calor, rubor, dolor et tumor. A fifth response, loss of function, is often present – a sprained ankle, for example, won't let you walk on it.

At a microscopic level, there's shedloads of stuff going on, with different sorts of white cells, chemicals, enzymes, antibodies and Lord knows what else doing their own thing, allied to enough intrinsic complexity for biochemists to make a whole career out of it, and pharmaceutical companies lots of money developing drugs to quash it. (The original anti-inflammatory medication is willow tree bark, though the active ingredient, salicin, was eventually synthesised as acetylsalicylic acid, otherwise known as aspirin.)

For our purposes, the simple hot, red, painful, swelling description will do, because to fully appreciate bellyache, you need to understand inflammation of the peritoneum, or peritonitis. Hang on, that sounds a bit lame. You need to understand – cue drumroll – peritonitis. That's better. It deserves a dramatic introduction.

What follows is a generic tale. It's true in every respect but garnered from hundreds of similar patients I've dealt with. Peritonitis is a common, but never routine, emergency.

A&E, three o'clock, Sunday morning. A fifty-year-old man with severe bellyache. The SHO tells me it's generalised, as opposed to localised peritonitis, with air under the diaphragm. I check the X-rays first, a chest and erect abdominal film. Sure enough, there's a telltale sliver of blackness under the dome of the diaphragm. Free air (or free flatus; fart) has no business in the abdomen. It's a catch-all green light for an emergency laparotomy. Something is perforated.

I find the man on a trolley in a curtained cubicle, wide-eyed with anxiety, sweaty and grey with pain; his lips have a tint of blue because of shallow breathing. He drags the oxygen mask from his face, 'Please don't feel my stomach,' he whispers, 'It hurts too much.'

'Don't worry, I don't need to, but ...' I show him my stethoscope, 'do you mind if I just have a quick listen?' It's a neat trick, particularly in kids. Placing the business end on his belly, with a little pressure I can feel it's as stiff as a board, which serves my purpose. Out of curiosity, I also have a listen. As expected, there are no gurgling bowel sounds. The abdomen is silent.

'When did this happen?'

'About midnight. Felt like I'd been shot. Now it's on fire.'

'Ever get indigestion?'

'Sometimes I take a Rennie tablet.'

'You need an operation. I'll see you again soon, upstairs.'

The peritoneum is a thin film of tissue lining everything inside the abdomen. It's as if a lunatic decorator has walked into your living room and sprayed it all red. The walls, the carpeted floor, ceiling, doors, windows, and all the furniture, sofa, chairs, coffee table, TV, stereo, radiators, bookcase. Absolutely everything that's red is peritoneum. In this analogy the walls, floor and ceiling are the abdominal wall, and the furniture all the assorted organs. To get you orientated, the light fitting in the middle of the ceiling is the "inside" aspect of your belly button, and out of view, just above the ceiling, is your six-pack of muscle and then skin.

The internal organs – the furniture – have the primeval visceral nerve supply which we inherited from that sea cucumber, but nonetheless does an adequate job. So, what nerves supply the peritoneum of the walls, floor and ceiling – the abdominal wall? It's those same highly specific skin nerves, so sensitive they can tell a pin prick from a tickle with a feather. Learned doctors and anatomists call them parietal nerves from *pariet*, (which, would you believe it, is Latin for wall.) The parietal nerves aren't quite as abundant and sensitive as those in your fingertips or lips, but they're much better than visceral nerves. Three billion years of evolution better.

Now, let's get back to our man with generalised peritonitis. Every part of the peritoneum inside his belly is inflamed, which is why I had the lunatic decorator use red paint. That is, it's hot, red, painful and swollen. The surface area of the peritoneum is roughly the same as our skin, so in effect he has the equivalent of total body sunburn, or worse, a scald. A one hundred percent skin scald. It's a massive injury.

All the visceral and parietal nerves are screaming in anguish. Moving, even breathing, is agony, so he lays quite still, taking rapid shallow breaths using only his ribcage rather than his diaphragm, which is held stiff and rigid.

Consequently, his oxygen levels plummet and his lips go blue. (*Note the difference to colic where patients squirm, curl up, or walk about, taking deep breaths with every paroxysm of pain. Just like a woman in labour, with her bright red well-oxygenated face. It's remarkable how we are all hardwired to respond similarly to different types of pain. Good clinicians will immediately recognise such clues.*)

His belly is so sensitive he can almost feel approaching footsteps. A careless kick to the trolley he's on is torture, and someone pressing his abdomen to palpate it would be excruciating, so he holds those muscles stiff also. His abdomen exhibits board-like rigidity.

The peritoneum is too thin to really swell, but instead it weeps inflammatory fluid, litres of it, resulting in dehydration, a falling blood pressure and a rapid pulse. The inflammation is so severe the gut becomes flaccid and immobile – loss of function – so his abdomen has no gurgles to hear. It is silent.

Untreated, he'd be dead within a day or two.

An hour or so later, after rapid fluid resuscitation and diamorphine (heroin) for the pain, he's anaesthetised and on the operating table. The resuscitation is important, without it he'd crash and burn from the anaesthetic. A short midline incision to start with, it can always be extended upwards or downwards depending on what's found. There's a puff of gas as the peritoneum is opened, but it doesn't smell of fart, which is relatively good news. Now, the incision is big enough to peer inside and I can see peas and chewed chips floating about in a sea of grey gunk, probably a mixture of tea and fish. I remember an Irishman, years earlier, brought in straight from a pub with six pints of Guinness sloshing about his insides. By the time I'd finished, the theatre smelt like a brewery.

I extend the incision north rather than south, thankful it'll be a perforated duodenal ulcer (perf DU) rather than the colon leaking shit: that could take hours and stinks so badly you'd gag and chew on it. Sure enough, there it is, a one-centimetre hole in the front of the duodenum, leaking green bile and stomach acid strong enough to etch metal. No wonder it's so painful. A few stitches to close the hole, reinforced with a patch of nearby fatty tissue. Job done. Wash out the fish supper with litres of warm saline (stand back or you'll soak your pants), check every nook and cranny for errant chips or peas, wash out again, then close up.

Post-op, he'll need a drip and suck regime for a few days because his bowel won't be functioning, plus prophylactic antibiotics, and whatever is flavour of the month to treat his ulcer. Discharge home after a week, six-week out-patient follow-up, then he can get on with his life.

One in twelve people reading this will have suffered appendicitis, the most common abdominal emergency. If you've never had it, you're still in with a chance, so it might be useful to describe the common symptoms using your newfound bellyache diagnostic skills. They could come in handy one day, particularly since appendicitis has an overall 1% mortality rate. What? Surely not; it's a minor inconvenience isn't it, like having a painful tooth pulled? The answer to both is no. It's potentially lethal, though the infirm elderly and immature young are most at risk. That's why appendicectomy (or appendectomy in the US) has been the treatment of choice for well over a hundred years, despite the risks of anaesthesia and surgery way back then. So, read carefully and Nota Bene as one of my schoolmasters was fond of saying.

Appendix derives from the Latin, to append, and humans have at least three places where the word is used to describe an "add-on" anatomic feature – the larynx, the testicles (*yes, really*), and the one we are interested in, which is found at the beginning of the colon or large bowel. Anatomists call it the vermiform (worm-like) appendix to avoid confusion. The length of your little finger and the width of a garden worm, it's another cul-de-sac diverticulum, and the remnant of a much larger structure our distant ancestors possessed when lazing around the tropical jungle, grooming each other's fur for fleas and ticks, chewing on vegetation, and dreaming of evolution. Back then, it helped to digest plant cellulose, but now serves as a sanctuary and reservoir of friendly colonic bacteria for when the rest of the colonic population is wiped out by a hostile infection like dysentery. The downside is, being so long and narrow makes it prone to obstruction and infection.

So firstly, appendicitis is an –itis, telling us the appendix is inflamed due to infection. Secondly, it's a midgut structure with a primitive visceral nerve supply. Both of these facts translate into a vague continuous pain around the belly button.

The appendix sits in the right lower abdomen, quite near that iliac bone you can feel with your right hand, just above your belt. Or, to go back to the living room analogy, it's the TV sitting in the right-hand corner next to the fireplace. If the infection and inflammation (red paint) spreads from the appendix (TV), it will involve the peritoneum in that corner of the abdominal (living room) wall. Those sensitive parietal nerves now tell you there's localized peritonitis in that area, and it really starts to hurt, seemingly shifting the pain from around the belly button to the right lower quadrant. The visceral nerves are still transmitting, but the signal is poor compared to the high fidelity attention-grabbing parietal ones.

Movement causes pain so you minimize it. A prod in that area is akin to poking a boil on the skin, so the muscles are held taut to protect the underlying inflammation from further prodding and pain – so-called guarding. But the canny doctor doesn't prod you there; instead he presses slowly and deeply on the opposite side, where it doesn't hurt, and then suddenly releases the pressure. The shock wave travels across the abdomen to produce "rebound" tenderness and you yelp with pain.

Now's the time to get your appendix removed, because if the infection continues to spread unfettered by the immune system, it could end up as generalised peritonitis, like the man with a perf DU, and kill you.

One elderly GP I knew didn't bother with all the tricksy diagnostic stuff. He simply asked the patient to stand on their right leg and jump up and down a few times, which I suppose is one way to jiggle up a tender appendix. His referral letters were terse:

"Appendicitis. Hop test positive. Please treat."

So, feel free to ignore everything I've taught you, and hop it.

For personal reasons, which I'll come to, this tutorial on bellyache wouldn't be complete without mention of the kidneys and the ureters. To recap, the kidneys in the loins produce urine, which is transported to the bladder via their respective ureters, and both lay at the back of the abdomen behind the peritoneum – in effect, beneath the fitted carpet on the floor of our notional living room. This means they are sandwiched between the extremely sensitive parietal nerves in the back wall of the abdomen, and the non-specific visceral nerves of the peritoneum in front, and have a unique dual nerve supply.

So what? Well, pain from the kidney and ureter is felt mainly in the loin and flank of the appropriate side, rather than the usual visceral abdominal midline. Pain is most commonly caused by a small stone from the kidney being squeezed along the squirming worm-like ureter. Once the stone is pushed into the bladder, the pain stops, and the stone is eventually peed out. Renal colic, or more correctly ureteric colic, is so overwhelmingly agonising it will reduce grown men – like me – to tearful puking wimps. It really is that awful.

As in gut colic, it's caused by the muscle of the ureter having to work so hard to push the stone along that it cramps up and goes into spasm. But the pain is far more severe because much of it is transmitted by the sensitive parietal nerves arising from the spinal cord, rather than the less-sensitive visceral nerves. What's more, the brain interprets the signal not as pain from the kidney and ureter, but from the areas of skin those same nerves supply – so-called referred pain. The griping pain, therefore, is felt in waves from the loin to the groin, and is reliably diagnostic of ureteric colic. It's pure luck the pain only extends down as far as the groin, since that area of skin represents the lowest nerve root the ureter has contact with before entering the bladder. If the ureter was an inch or two longer, it's quite feasible the pain of ureteric colic would be picked up by lower spinal nerve roots, and consequently be felt from the loin all the way down to the knee or ankle. Wouldn't that be odd? And oh boy, wouldn't it confuse the orthopods?

I suffered a kidney stone a few years after retirement, so had no instant access to friendly colleagues in my own hospital. Armed with a self-diagnosis, some idea of how the system works, and in great distress, I presented in the early hours of the morning to the triage nurse of nearest A&E department. 'Hello (*groan*), I've got left ureteric colic (*gasp*). And no, I'm not a junkie and I'm not (*grunt*) trying to blag some pethidine.'

'Crikey, Grandad, how old are you? We stopped falling for that one years ago. These days, you get a diclofenac suppository. Want one?'

'Yes please. Hand it over now and I'll insert it myself. Better still, give me two.'

12

KNIFE AND DEATH

"We want you to do everything possible to save our mum. Even if the operation kills her, she should have that chance. You won't do it 'cos she's old. It's all about saving money, isn't it? You've at least got to try. We'll pay to go private."

Every surgeon regularly faces such demands and accusations, often from a group of hostile siblings motivated by a mixture of fear, unrealistic expectations, and a sudden realisation that time is running out for their loved one. Most adults go through the same guilt-trip when an elderly parent is facing the inevitable. Busy lives, young children and demanding jobs mean any broken promises will come back to haunt you, no matter how caring and thoughtful you've been through the years. So, the siblings decide, now's the time to make amends for all those perceived failings by leaning on the surgeon and throwing some weight about. Usually, mum is frail, well past her best-before date, at death's door with a gangrenous leg or whatever else is killing her, and needs sympathetic terminal care rather than surgery. Or, for example, she has troublesome gallstones and is rather enjoying the newfound attention they bring, but is also obese, with heart failure, terrible lungs, turns blue and breathless if she thinks too hard, can't lay flat, is wheelchair bound, on piped oxygen, and isn't fit enough for a haircut, let alone an operation.

Whichever the case, the conversation goes something like this:

'If I operate on her, I'll kill her.'

'We're willing to take that risk and so is she.'

'You're not listening to me. It is not a *risk*. She *will* die.'

'You *can't* know that for sure.'

'I can. And I do.'

'If she was *your* mum, you'd operate.'

'No, I wouldn't. And I'd stop anyone else from doing so.'

What follows next is a threat. I must agree to operate or find another surgeon who will, otherwise they'll complain to the press, the hospital management, the GMC, and their member of parliament. '… And you won't like that, will you?'

Unless the psychiatric unit has one locked up in a padded cell, I know for sure there won't be another surgeon lunatic enough to go anywhere near their mum, but I eventually learned to sidestep the aggressive standoff by playing my trump card first. 'Tell you what, let's get a second opinion from an anaesthetist. After all, if no one's prepared to put her to sleep, she can't have an operation.'

The anaesthetist sees the patient and then speaks to the family: 'There's absolutely no need for you to worry about your mum surviving an operation. The anaesthetic alone will kill her.'

Anaesthetists are even more pessimistic than surgeons, and since neither of us enjoy killing people, we do our best to avoid it.

At the other end of the fitness-for-operation spectrum are young adults who can generally survive any surgery required. Most patients, obviously, lie somewhere in between and need appropriate individual consideration. Children have their own set of rules because they are not simply small people, but completely different bundles of grief with an immature body, physiology and immune system, and will release their tenuous grip on life at the slightest opportunity.

All of which leads to the question you've always longed to ask of a surgeon, but never dared. 'How many patients have you legally killed with a knife?' The easy answer is that every operation I've ever done has a 100% mortality – eventually. Now you say, 'No, that's not what I meant. Instead, tell me how many patients have you killed by cutting the wrong thing by mistake?' That's easy as well. I've never cut anything by mistake because my mind has already cut, incised or divided it five minutes before my hand does. If I cut that, will there be bleeding I can or can't control? Could it kill the patient or make them worse or better than they already are? Can I repair any damage caused for the greater benefit? As a young man with little experience I wasn't as assured as I am now, but years of practice and a thorough knowledge of anatomy helps, as does not being scared shitless by bleeding. 'Dammit,' you say, 'How many of your patients died on the table or soon after?' Well, that's a much better question, and the answer is, unfortunately, quite a few.

There are some conditions – leaking aneurysms, deadly knife or firearm wounds, severe trauma, gangrene of the whole gut, rampant peritonitis or cancer – that surgery can't salvage even though they demand an attempt; the degree of damage, sepsis or pathology being irretrievable and incompatible with life. And sadly, there were some patients who proved to be too sick or too old to withstand surgery, but I made the mistake of trying anyway. As I became older and wiser there were fewer of them, but those errors still weigh on my conscience. Then again, some patients didn't get their operation soon enough because I thought they were improving without surgery. More mistakes.

In truth, and to be a little more serious, slip-of-hand errors are rare unless the anatomy is grossly distorted by, for example, large tumours. The majority of surgical mistakes prove to be of timing or decision-making, but can only be recognised as such with hindsight, or, as we say, through the retrospectoscope. A common scenario is the patient who is slow to recover from bowel surgery. Is there a leak at the anastomosis, a twist in the bowel, a bleed, a diminished blood supply? Should I re-operate or not, do it now or wait a little longer, get another investigation first? When in doubt, absolutely the easiest option is to dive back in, but if nothing remiss is found the patient can be harmed or their recovery seriously setback for no reason. Waiting too long and then finding something that should have been fixed earlier is an equally depressing guilt-ridden torment. My yardstick has generally been sleep: will I sleep tonight if I don't operate today? Or, I didn't sleep last night, so I'll do it this morning if there's been no improvement. One surgeon I know made such worrisome decisions in the Blackwall Tunnel during his daily commute. He called them his 'BT patients.'

A classic 'slip of hand' is cutting a ureter – the tube carrying urine from the kidney to bladder – and has been covered in a previous chapter. Gynaecologists are the usual culprits.

Another classic is cutting the common bile duct – the tube carrying bile from the liver to the gut – and happens during gallbladder removal for painful stones. Both structures are intimately related, so need careful dissection and positive identification of the anatomy before the gallbladder can be safely excised. Failure to do so correctly is possibly the worst error a general surgeon can commit, and causes all sorts of grief for the patient. Though not necessarily deadly, damage to the common bile duct – even after being repaired – will often blight a patient's health for life, as it did for Anthony Eden, a former British prime minister.

Happily, I've never cut a ureter or a common bile duct in error. But some deaths, and some misdeeds, will stay with me forever.

Tuesday afternoon, an operating list full of inguinal (Latin: *inguin*; groin) hernia repairs in the hospital's Day Unit. It's a common problem in men because they carry their gonads

– testicles – outside the abdomen and consequently have weak groins where the spermatic cord, which arises within the abdomen, pierces through the muscle layers to enter the scrotum. The weak area allows protrusions of fat or intestine to bulge into the groin and cause an abnormal swelling called a hernia, or in some parts of the country, "A nernia." Since women keep their gonads – ovaries – safely and wisely tucked away on the inside, they only rarely suffer the same complaint. As a consultant, I repaired about 250 groin hernias in men each year, and many thousands throughout my career, all without significant incident. Except one.

It was no different to countless other day-case lists. Five or six instantly forgettable fit men on a virtual conveyor belt, expertly anaesthetised by a senior consultant, with a turnaround time for each patient of about thirty minutes. By five-thirty I was doing a post-op ward round to check all was well, and dispensing sundry advice to each patient before they were discharged home. One man had just finished his complimentary cup of tea and was sitting up, comfortably relaxed on his trolley. A junior nurse was collecting the cup and asking if he'd like a refill, though she stepped to one side when I entered the curtained-off cubicle. He turned his attention to me and smiled.

'Hi, just popping by to say the operation was straightforward with no problems. Your groin is now reinforced with mesh, so you shouldn't have any further trouble. Take the pain killers regularly, just as it says on the packet, and don't–'

As I reeled off my patter his eyelids fell shut, his jaw fell slackly open, and his head lolled to one side. Unconscious, gone, out of it. A shake, a slap, a shout made no difference, nor did a heavy thump to his chest with my fist. I didn't bother checking anything else. Punching the red emergency button on the wall behind him set various klaxons hooting throughout the unit, and together with the nurse, we ran the man's trolley back to the theatre recovery room, shouting for help as we went. In less than half a minute, he was getting first-class cardio-pulmonary resuscitation from a bunch of anaesthetists and technicians within the department, and they were quickly joined by the hospital "Crash" team. Continuous external cardiac massage, tracheal intubation with oxygen, electrocardiogram monitor, defibrillation shocks, intravenous adrenaline and other drugs, the whole shebang orchestrated by my ITU-trained anaesthetist and the cardiologist in the crash team, and all done with the calm professionalism and ruthless urgency portrayed in the movies and TV soaps. But this was for real, went on for an hour, and the guy didn't make it. Fixed dilated pupils put an end to proceedings.

'Who's supposed to be collecting him?' I asked the Day Unit sister.

We were in her office along with an older woman in a smart charcoal suit, the on-call hospital manager, who also happened to be the senior nursing officer, formerly known as matron. Both were good at their jobs. 'It's his wife …' Sister eyed the fob-watch pinned to her breast pocket, 'and she'll be expecting a call to come and get him anytime now.'

It was close on seven. Outside the office window it was already dark, with a steady dismal drizzle. 'That can't happen. We can't tell a wife that her husband's dead over the bloody phone. It has to be face-to-face. Gimme the address and I'll go there now, before she gets anxious and rings us.' Rising from my chair, I was already composing the script in my head, and would fine-tune it on the way. Purveying terrible news is always the consultant's job. I'd done it often enough, though never for a simple hernia.

The manager lifted her pensive gaze from the floor, suddenly animated, 'NO. It can't be you. You're too involved with the case. And on your own, a strange man, to a young woman's house, at night? It's a recipe for … well, for any number of things, and they're all bad. I won't allow it.' She shook her head for emphasis.

'You come with me then, as chaperone.'

'I said, no. And with or without me, it's still no because somehow it doesn't feel right. One of us will do it. In fact, we'll both go, there are probably children to consider and we'll be of more use.' Both women nodded to each other in agreement.

I slumped back into my seat, forced there by some feminine intuition beyond my understanding, or maybe they were simply protecting me from a frenzied attack by a distraught wife. 'Okay, but get going now, and hurry. I'll get things organised at this end.'

With them gone, I picked up the desk phone and asked the switchboard to get hold of the coroner's officer. They're invariably retired police officers, always helpful, hugely knowledgeable and very efficient. 'Hello there, long time no see. What can I do you for?' And totally predictable.

'Hi, Paul. Sorry to bother you at this hour. It's a forty-year-old man with a wife and presumed kids. Unexpected post-op death following a hernia repair I did this afternoon. We crashed him for a good hour but couldn't get him going. He'll need a coroner's PM for cause of death. At present, he's in the Day Unit but they'll move him to the mortuary any time soon …'

After relaying the patient's details, I wandered back to the recovery suite to ensure everything was ready for the transfer. All the debris from earlier had been cleaned away and it was deserted, except for the body under a white sheet, and the same tea-toting junior nurse sitting guard next to it, the thin file of notes clasped firmly to her chest beneath folded arms. She looked no older than my just-teenaged daughter, yet seemed fully at ease rather than spooked. My raised eyebrows asked the obvious question.

'I've been told to sit with him until the porters come to take him away.' Her easy manner told me she didn't have a clue who I was. Either that, or she hadn't yet been told never to speak to consultants.

'That's good of you,' I smiled.

'I don't mind. He was a nice man. Since you're here, do you know if it would be okay to open a window?'

'Why, are you too hot?'

'No, I'm fine. It's just that my nan says you should always open a window so the spirit can escape.' By way of explanation, she added, 'She was a nurse too. A long time ago.'

'Well, if that's what your nan says, we'd better do it.' I knew it to be an old nursing tradition, so went to the nearest frosted pane and duly obliged. 'Is that wide enough? Any more will let the rain in.'

'That should do. Thanks.'

As a surgeon, it's an inescapable fact that some patients will die as a direct or indirect result of your actions. I'm sure each of us has our own way of reconciling the dilemma, other than giving up completely. For me, knowing how or why a patient died is important, because it permits or denies the forgiveness my conscience yearns for. A routine aneurysm repair who dies from a heart attack three weeks after a full recovery would be absolved, though I would regret ever doing the operation. One who bled to death after three days because a suture gave way would fill me with guilt, make me doubt my ability, and could never be forgiven. In both cases, knowing the cause of death provides a resolution of sorts, and a determination to do better. Not knowing is purgatory.

Driving home through that filthy night, I couldn't help but ponder what killed my hernia man, and a rare but familiar anxiety gripped tighter with each rhythmic beat of the windscreen wipers. Guilt, doubt, guilt, doubt …

Pulmonary embolus – PE, a blood clot in the lungs – was the consensus view, but it didn't sit well with me. The clot comes from leg veins after a deep vein thrombosis (DVT) in people immobilised by illness, a prolonged operation, a long-haul flight, or women on the Pill. He didn't fit the bill. And the manager in me was obsessive about DVT prevention, even for day cases. 'I don't care if every patient in the whole bloody hospital drops dead tomorrow with a PE. As long as they do it wearing stockings and on heparin, we can't be held negligent,' was my usual broadside to errant colleagues. And yet, it was a possibility. Guilt, doubt, guilt, doubt …

I fumbled a cigarette to my lips and lit it, then cracked open a window to draw the smoke away, but my brain wouldn't stop grinding. My money was on a massive heart attack or stroke, but he could have bled to death from something I damaged and didn't notice – there are some big blood vessels deep in the groin. Whatever the cause, he died at the point of my knife. Guilt, doubt, guilt, doubt …

Depressing and alarming, but shit happens, usually when it's least expected. And what's done is done. I knew to ignore the misgivings, put the "what-ifs" to one side, shrug off the brooding unease. Or bottle it up, at least until the facts emerged. To do otherwise would lead to madness. Since it was out of my hands, I resolved to try not to think about it. The post-mortem would sort it. Show the how and the why. Or put me in the frame. Guilt, doubt, guilt, doubt …

After a fitful sleep, the coroner's officer rang me the following day, at the end of the morning's aneurysm. 'The PM's booked for tomorrow lunchtime. Under the circumstances, rather than any of your pathologists doing it, the coroner wants an independent Home Office one. It's so the family or any lawyers can't point a finger and complain about collusion. Not unusual.'

'Okay, Paul, got that. Now, tell me, are there any legal

objections to me watching it?'

'No, none at all. Fill your boots.'

When a patient dies, the attending doctor has a legal duty to truthfully record the primary cause of death, and any contributing causes, on a death certificate. As in: *Bled to death; Massive trauma; Run over by a bus.* But it's not always so easy: *Possible brain secondaries; Presumed ovarian cancer*, just won't do. Nor will: *Stopped breathing*.

Forty years ago, before the advent of sophisticated body scanners which visualise almost any pathology in the living, post-mortems were a daily event in every hospital to establish cause of death if it wasn't obvious or known. Only then could the death certificate be accurately completed. As a student, the teaching hospital pathologists held classes in the mortuary every weekday at noon to demonstrate all the noteworthy diseases found in that morning's line up of corpses – an unwholesome, often smelly, yet unforgettable visual and tactile education, which has all but gone. These days PMs are still done, but primarily for deaths that are suspicious or have an unknown cause. My man ticked both boxes.

And so, on that Thursday, after the clinic and ward round, I led the juniors and three medical students into what was for them, the unknown territory of the mortuary and PM room. The senior technician answered the bell and unlocked the heavy door to welcome us in.

'Hello there, I knew you'd come. And I see you've brought the young 'uns with you.' Short, bald and round, with theatre greens stretched tight over his belly, his old creased face always beamed enthusiasm. He was happy in his job, and happier still when visitors came.

'If that's okay with you, Nev. I think it'll do them good to see what you get up to in here.'

'Course it is. Come in, come in.'

Neville handed out blue theatre hats and paper gowns to wear over our clothes, led us along yards of twisting corridors, then fussily arranged us in a line on one side of the PM room. 'You'll be safe here, away from any splashes, but close enough to see.'

The naked body of my patient dominated centre stage, with an array of overhead lights brightly illuminating the scene. He lay on a ribbed stainless-steel table, little more than an overly long draining board, with a bucket positioned beneath the drain hole between his ankles. His head was propped up on a brown wooden block, eyelids not quite shut, with the neat thin line of my hernia incision sitting accusingly in his left groin. On a tray at the foot of the table were various knives and instruments, and nearby, other trays and tables held power saws, bowls, jugs, cutting blocks and weighing scales. Several deep sinks and work surfaces lined one wall, and above them hung a large blackboard marked in a grid of painted lines with a list of organs printed along the left-hand edge, for recording weights and other features: brain, liver, lungs, kidneys …

In short, a temple dedicated to the spotless utility of stainless steel and white ceramic tiles. Or the back room of a butcher's shop.

Promptly, at one o'clock, we heard the distant doorbell at the locked entrance ring, and soon afterwards, a beaming Neville reverentially escorted the visiting pathologist through the door. Her startling appearance drew a muted gasp from my small group. It was Morticia Addams from *The Addams Family*.

Tall and slim, long straight jet-black hair with a central parting, a pale complexion accentuated by darkly shaded mascara, with a slash of red at her lips, she was dressed entirely in funereal black: shoes, tights, knee-length pencil skirt and tailored five-button jacket, save for a short V of white blouse beneath her neck. At once imperious, attractive, and in the context, shockingly macabre, she looked to be in her mid to late thirties and radiated absolute command and control. Marching the few steps in my direction, she shook my hand, 'Hi, I've read the brief. Let me get changed and we'll get started.'

Ten minutes later, she was standing at the table in a theatre gown and hat, white boots, surgical mask, protective eye goggles, full-length brown rubber apron, and heavy-duty elbow-length red gloves. Neville was on the opposite side, similarly attired. 'THE BODY IS THAT OF A WELL-NOURISHED WHITE MALE …' she began. My entourage glanced quizzically at me. I pointed to the thin wire with a tiny microphone hanging from one of the overhead lights and whispered, 'It's all being recorded.' An hour later, with the body totally eviscerated, all organs weighed and salami sliced, including the brain, she finally held the heart up to the light in her left hand, and once again used a thin long carving knife to slice quick multiple cuts across the coronary arteries and into the underlying muscle, each time examining the cut surface in minute detail. '… NO EVIDENCE OF CORONARY OR MYOCARDIAL DISEASE.' Then she plonked the heart onto an empty scale, carefully placed the knife on a tray and walked towards me, gloved hands clasped together at her waist.

'I can't find anything, and I can't tell you why he died. The toxicology screen will take a few days and I'll send the heart off to a cardiac pathologist, which will take even longer. For now, that's all I'm able to say.'

Two or three months down the line and I was sitting in a coroner's court, the back row occupied by journalists with notepads looking for a story, the front row occupied by a large family with grim faces looking for answers. Witnesses and representatives of all interested parties, including the hospital legal team, were scattered in between. It was quite a turn out. All the previous ones I had attended – it's an infrequent part of the job – were held around a single table and numbered fewer than a decent-sized dinner party. It began, as ever, with the lady coroner stating the purpose of the gathering. 'To ascertain the cause of death, and not to apportion blame.'

I wasn't called as a witness. The coroner could see no purpose in asking the surgeon (*a simple, thick, surgeon?*) to assist the court, given that a perfectly routine and flawless hernia repair coincided with the man's death. With a puff of my cheeks, I agreed with her wholeheartedly. My anaesthetist chum was called, and recounted the standard anaesthetic and

CPR attempt, including the provision of some remarkably clever drugs and chemicals, most of which went way over my head.

I didn't spot Morticia in the crowd of heads until the coroner called her to the stand. Once again, she was a vision in black, wearing exactly the same outfit as before. From a distance, the flash of white blouse at her throat resembled a barrister's jabot, or court bib, and finally explained both her ensemble and the reason for it. Half her job entailed regularly appearing in court as an expert witness, the other half gathering evidence by doing post-mortems, and likely doing both on the same day. Since suitably respectful attire is required when attending every type of court, criminal or otherwise, her sombre garb was a rational daily necessity rather than some wilful fashion statement. Case solved.

She gave an in-depth account of how the post-mortem and a host of erudite super-specialists had helped her reach a decision regarding my man's cause of death. And that was – wait for it – she didn't know. No abnormality, nothing, zip, zilch, could be found at the PM, or by any of the additional forensic investigations.

'How many post-mortems do you undertake each year?' the coroner asked.

'Over eight hundred.'

'And of that number, how often do you find no cause of death?'

'Less than fifty.'

My first reaction was, *WOW*. Over eight hundred PMs a

year amounted to the equivalent of three or more major operations every working day. The subjects don't need a time-consuming anaesthetic, or to survive her ministrations, but it was still a huge number. My second reaction was sadness and disappointment. Sadness for the man, his family, their lost future together, and disappointment that none of us would ever truly know why he died. Nevertheless, I was off the hook, as was my anaesthetist. We had both guessed as much after the initial PM, so it came as no surprise, despite the many weeks of niggling anxiety.

Sudden unexplained death of young adults accounts for the 5%, or thereabouts, of negative post-mortems reported by forensic experts like Morticia. And remember, they only do the suspicious ones, or those with no known cause, so the overall number is tiny compared to deaths as a whole. Yet the social, financial and psychological misery they cause to affected families is disproportionately huge. Sudden arrhythmic death syndrome, or SADS – a rather appropriate acronym for a heart that simply stops beating – causes about 500 deaths a year in the UK out of a grand total of 600,000, and is probably what killed my man. Screening is now available for people with a family history.

I once dived into the belly of a seventy-year-old man with a leaking aortic aneurysm – nothing unusual in that – but it turned out to be one of those few operations you wish you had never started. It was the usual middle-of-the-night scramble of urgency, blood, more blood and structured panic, ably assisted by Roy Orbison and the rest of the team. After perhaps two hours of taxing hard work, the problem was fixed with an implanted Dacron graft and all had gone well. It was time to sew him up. Whilst wrestling the gut back into some sort of anatomical order within the abdomen, I felt a golf ball-size lump in the lower end of his stomach. Closer inspection showed white seedlings, like dozens of tiny pearls, blossoming through to the external surface of the stomach wall. It was cancer, previously undiagnosed, yet already at an advanced stage. *Shit.* Even with no eyeball evidence of spread elsewhere, there would be countless other microscopic seedlings throughout the abdominal cavity and in his liver. Before too long they would grow, fill his belly with malignant fluid, and overwhelm him. If he survived the aneurysm repair, a lingering death from cancer awaited, a calamity brought about by my own unwitting hand.

Had I known of the advanced cancer pre-operatively, without any qualms or fear of reprisal, I would have refused to do the operation, of that I'm certain. He would have been given morphine for pain and allowed to bleed to death very quickly. Once inside his belly, if I had discovered the cancer before tackling the aneurysm, as I should have, I'm not sure what I would have done. Seek guidance from his wife and children? No time for that, and probably grossly unfair to ask. Carry on regardless? Possibly. But, thankfully, that conundrum never arose. The deed was already done. To prevent the cancer obstructing his stomach and causing death by vomiting, starvation and dehydration, I removed it with a wide margin and plumbed the much smaller stomach remnant back into continuity with the bowel; a palliative service only, but one I felt duty-bound to provide. Only chemotherapy might help him thereafter. Unfortunately, in my opinion, he made a full recovery and was passed over to the cancer specialists.

Perhaps I allowed him some extended time to write a will, put his affairs in order, and make peace with family and friends, but it's the only solace I have. I'm not sure any good work was done that night. What life he had remaining would have been short and miserable, made worse by chemotherapy, and a dawning realisation the aneurysm was a preferable exit route. It would have been a bad death. The leaking aneurysm would have been a good one.

I've no idea of a layman's perception of a good death. Something out of Hollywood perhaps, with music, clean sheets, plumped pillows, lots of hand-holding, fond goodbyes, no regrets, heavy eyelids followed by gentle sleep and a long final sigh. For experienced medics and anyone who knows the excruciating agony of watching a loved one suffer as they die, a good death requires no pain, no anxiety, no frightening breathlessness, no drowning sensation, no nausea or vomiting, no bedsores, and no humiliating incontinence. Anything else is peripheral window dressing. Sadly, it's all too rare. A good death requires fearless nursing and large doses of opiates (heroin, morphine) at the very least, and in my case will be supplemented with single malt

Scotch whisky; east coast please, the west coast peaty stuff tastes like cough medicine. A bad death is the converse of good and is generally caused by well-meaning carers not being liberal enough with the morphine. The word is derived from *Morpheus,* the Roman god of sleep, so there's your clue. If I'm not asleep or drowsy – and most importantly, pain free – up the morphine until I am. It will not turn me into a hippie-cum-junkie, nor will it kill me, the underlying terminal illness is already doing that. Morphine will make me insensate to any nastiness and allow my body to wave a white flag and surrender.

There is no poetry in death. It is ugly, brutal, painful and shitty, as is birth. I delivered forty babies as a student, and have witnessed many more deaths, so speak from experience. I have no memory of being born, and similarly, no wish to be aware of dying. Any poetic nonsense arises from the hearts and minds of onlookers, or worse, the arty imagination of those with absolutely no knowledge of it. A peaceful comfortable death is resolutely to go gentle into that good night. Should I feel the urge to rage, rage against the dying of the light, I'll do it while I still have my wits, and well before I'm on my death bed. It is noteworthy that Dylan Thomas was in a coma and on a ventilator when he died.

Dennis Potter, the famous British dramatist and screenwriter, did a television interview in 1994, three months before he died from pancreatic cancer. I remember seeing it and admiring his courageous common sense. Throughout the lengthy conversation he quaffed a champagne and morphine concoction of his own formulation, which kept him pleasantly pain free, completely lucid, totally in control, and, he explained, allowed him to continue writing in order to finish off a few projects before he made his exit. Way to go, Dennis.

Of course, I can always hope to drop down dead from a massive heart attack, stroke, leaking aneurysm (would that be poetic justice?) or runaway truck. At least it'll be quick and clean. Whichever is destined for you, and I guarantee it will come, please sort out your will and affairs beforehand. With the modern fluid complexity of marriages, partnerships and parenthood, I've seen far too many bereaved people thrown into transient or permanent impoverishment, all for want of some simple pre-mortem organisation and planning.

Finally, spare a thought for the doctor who comes with bad tidings.

It was a boy aged five, brought into A&E after being hit by a car, and I was on call. 'Could you come and see if anything can be done?' An odd request, from a nurse, relayed over the phone and laced with foreboding. The child was in the resus room, lying on a soggy mess of bloody clothes that had clearly been hastily torn and scissored from his body. Both ankles had cut-down IV lines with O-neg blood pouring in, and the wall mounted heart monitor bleeped a miserably slow 50 as the trace crept across its screen. Not good. The trolley was surrounded by the half-dozen trauma team, each wearing their identification bib, each gloomily silent and strangely inactive. At the head end, an anaesthetist was hand-ventilating the boy's lungs, regularly squeezing the green reservoir balloon attached to the endo-tracheal breathing tube, a technique known as "bagging". Running across the child's right abdomen and lower chest was a twelve-inch ragged tear, and with each compression of the bag, foamy rivers of lurid red and green bubbled through the wound.

'What's up, Jay?' I asked the young consultant in charge.

'We can't keep up with the blood loss and wondered if you could stop whatever's bleeding. A second opinion if you like.' His defeated look told me all I needed to know.

Then, turning to the anaesthetist, another young man I knew from theatres, 'Is he anaesthetised or unconscious?'

'Oxygen only. Out of it since he arrived.'

With a gloved hand I explored the depths of the wound, forming an image in my mind's eye, and relayed it to the team. The liver was mashed to pulp. Immediately above it the right diaphragm had a wide split, allowing my probing fingers to enter the chest cavity and release a foaming gush of scarlet bubbles through to the wound – the lung was damaged and leaking oxygen. Further across the abdomen I felt a huge collection of fluid at the back, behind the peritoneum – blood from one or both shattered kidneys, and probably a fractured pancreas. On the left side, the spleen was in pieces. A finger on the aorta confirmed a barely palpable blood pressure and slow pulse. When I withdrew my hand a litre of watery blood followed, and the glove was covered in bits of food, green bile and brown faeces – disruption of the small and large bowel. 'It's hopeless; the injuries are too great. What are the pupils doing?'

'They've been up and down a few times already. Right now …' Jay briefly lifted the eyelids, 'they're dilated again.'

I pulled off my gloves and threw them onto the pile of trash under the trolley. 'The chest and abdomen have been crushed, presumably by the impact or a wheel running over him. The pressure ruptured the diaphragm and ripped his belly open. I'm surprised he made it this far.'

'It happened less than a mile away, and the paramedics got him here quickly.'

Probably too quickly. Another few minutes and he would have died at the roadside. 'Well, Jay, in my opinion the injuries are incompatible with life. The injury to the liver is enough on its own, without the rest of it.'

He reluctantly reached to the IV lines and turned them off. The anaesthetist followed suit and stopped ventilating the lungs. Jay muttered, 'Is everyone in agreement?' We all nodded in unison. It took a few minutes for the heart monitor to flatline. Jay did the appropriate checks before pronouncing time of death, and then dismissed his team. Now he turned to me, eyes red with suppressed tears. *Here it comes. The real reason I was called. He can't face the relatives.* 'His parents are in the family room …'

'Yeah, leave it to me, Jay. I'm the on-call surgeon. It's probably best if I do it.'

'Thanks.'

Grabbing the notes, I found a quiet corner with a windowsill to lean on, and wrote a clear and easily understood account of my findings and opinion. Comprehensive enough, I hoped, to satisfy the coroner and prevent yet another request to attend a hearing. Then, having memorised the boy's name, I found the A&E sister and asked her to accompany me to the family room. Outside the door, we paused for a brief glance at each other, '*Ready?*' Then I took a deep breath, turned the handle, and pushed.

The couple were sitting side by side, hand in hand on a powder-blue sofa, the whole room a fusion of matt neutral tones. In their mid-twenties and little more than kids themselves, their upturned faces were white with fear. He had been their first child.

'Hello, I'm one of the doct–' That's as far as I got with the introductions. Mum took one look at me, then at Sister, and started screaming.

13

A CONSULTANT JOB

As a trainee would-be consultant, one spends perhaps ten years or more as a junior: grinding through job after job; climbing the ladder of seniority rung by rung; exams, more exams; research; higher degrees; publications; a spell overseas maybe. And then, suddenly, it's all over. You fill in the forms, get them endorsed by your boss, and send them off to whichever authority wields the rubber stamp for your specialty. Sometime later a certificate arrives which says you are fully trained, and the General Medical Council amends your entry in the medical register to confirm that fact to the public at large. Wonderful. On paper, you're as qualified as any of your former chiefs, though nowhere near as experienced. But in fact, the only qualification you have is the right to apply for a consultant post. It doesn't mean you'll get one.

You may be surprised to learn an NHS consultant job, like marriage, is supposed to be for life. However, unlike marriage, there's no courting, no living together beforehand, no intimacy, no parents or lunatic siblings to meet, no way of discovering a skeleton in the closet or getting used to disgusting habits, and no possibility of saying, 'It's me, not you,' if you want to end the relationship before walking up the aisle. Getting a consultant appointment only to discover you're in a marriage from hell is tough luck, but you're pretty much stuck with it.

Similarly, the hospital's existing consultants and CEO, the other bride or groom, have no idea if they're about to employ Frankenstein's monster or his wife for the rest of their professional life. It's like blindfold speed dating with the vicar waiting in the wings, anxious to get on with a wedding ceremony, for better, for worse, until death or retirement do us part. Furthermore, since all the potential brides or grooms have legitimate wedding banns published in the form of completion-of-training certificates, the employer can't argue one candidate is better qualified than another. So, if Frankenstein's monster does apply for the job, he must be considered.

Once appointed as a consultant, the chances of moving to another hospital in the same role are slim to non-existent, however disenchanted and incompatible you and your colleagues feel. What institution would risk taking on an unhappy bunny from another hospital when it can get a new unsullied one off the production line? Conversely, it's nigh on impossible to sack Frankenstein's monster unless it's for proven gross negligence, incompetence or criminal activity, in which case the consultant's trainers, previous employers, the GMC and possibly the police get embroiled in what is always an unholy mess.

I've seen a few consultant surgeons simply resign and

leave within a few years of appointment. If you're thinking racism, sexism or homophobia, forget it. Within surgery it's all about ability. Those who can cut, and cut well, suffer no prejudice. Those who can't are usually in trouble: loss of confidence, inability to cope with pressure, mental breakdown, a spouse or family feeling neglected, homesickness, or general disillusionment with consultant life and its bureaucracy. One I know went off to live on a boat (independent means, I presume), another secured a job with the WHO in Geneva, others abandoned the NHS for private practice or simply returned home to their country of origin. But the vast majority remain cheerfully optimistic, rub along with each other through the highs and lows of any job or marriage, and most will even turn up for your funeral or retirement bash, whichever comes first.

So, how can any institution ensure they're about to employ the right chap or chapess who'll fit in, do a good job and not jump ship at the first hiccup or when the going gets tough? In truth they can't, at least not legitimately, because employment law guards against any form of discrimination. In my time, it was routine to hold a sherry party for short-listed candidates. Known as "trial by sherry", it was a small soiree to give all interested and any alcoholic consultants a free drink and a chance to meet their potential future colleague. Held a few days before the formal interview, it was usually preceded by a quick tour to show off the newest wards, radiology machines, theatres and the like, and then convened in the boardroom or postgrad centre, whichever was most plush. Once there, the candidates were plied with sherry and canapés while being individually interrogated by dozens of people they didn't know, and a few they did. Speed dating without the blindfolds.

Afterwards, the hopefuls would retire to the nearest pub for a post-mortem and a beer: 'Hey, did you meet that anaesthetist with the shaky hands and a squint? I wouldn't let him loose on a dog.' Meanwhile, back at base, the consultants unscrewed the gin bottle and sat around discussing their individual preferences: 'Didn't much fancy that tall chap, the one with the flat head and strange lumps each side of his neck. Did anyone else think his hands were too big? Or is he an orthopod who's applied for the wrong job by mistake?'

Trial by sherry has long gone, replaced by individual candidates making an appointment to look around the hospital, meet the CEO and glad-hand influential consultants. It amounts to the same thing and is more politically correct, but equally uncertain to produce a happy and fruitful partnership.

The best fit is if the aspiring consultant is working at the hospital or has worked there previously. Plan A, or better the devil you know, is self-explanatory. A love-love relationship is highly satisfactory for both sides and unlikely to be thwarted by any interloper. It's also beneficial for both parties if they hate each other, since the aspirant won't apply for the job and the hospital won't have to reject him; a net gain for both and a chance to look elsewhere. However, a love-hate set up is awkward, especially for an applicant who's rejected by his present or previous institution. Such unpleasantness is generally circumvented with a kindly word from a senior consultant; 'Don't bother applying old chap, we've someone else lined up. Let us all just assume you didn't fancy the job.'

Plan B is to ring a mate on the old boy network. I've previously outlined this approach when garnering information on potential trainees, but it works equally well for senior appointments. 'Hi Joe, I hear you have a girl looking for a consultant post. If you think she'll fit in here, we'd like to see her.' Or, 'Hi Joe, you're interviewing one of my lads on Friday. I've no idea who else you're seeing, but I can tell you he's a good bloke (or, a nasty little shite) and we'd dearly like to keep him here (get rid of the bastard), but presently we have no jobs (no wish to ruin your life).'

Plan C is do it by the book and let HR handle it all. Advertise, shortlist, interview and appoint the best of a group of unknown candidates on the day. In an independent capacity, I've been on the appointment panel for a few of these. Absolutely the best result is when no candidate is good enough to be offered the job, generally because the flattering portrait painted by their CV mutates under forensic verbal scrutiny into a canvas of Jackson Pollock's. Second best, is when one of the candidates is offered the job but refuses it on the grounds that having recognised the abysmal calibre of his fellow interviewees, that the hospital would even consider them indicates he'd be better off elsewhere. The lesson of Plan C is that poor planning produces piss-poor performance. It should only ever be actioned to rubber-stamp the outcome Plan A and/or Plan B has already procured.

The appointments committee or interview panel for a consultant post is a wondrous behemoth. The CEO (panel chairman); a board member (the chairman or non-exec); an HR person (to disallow improper questions and check the paperwork); a string of appropriate specialty consultants from within the hospital; an outside consultant representing the College (of surgeons, physicians, anaesthetists, etc.); a few others for no discernible reason; and finally, a woman in a big hat. The latter is some sort of local community representative (health, patient group) to demonstrate the hospital is "in-touch" with its neighbourhood. She is infamous for being uninformed and asking crass questions:

'Doctor, I see from your CV that you're not married.' *This, to an anaesthetist chum of mine.*

'No, ma'am, I'm not.'

'Mm, I see. Does that mean you're a homosexual?'

'No, but if it'll get me the job, I'm willing to try anything once.'

Another one:

'The waiting list for hip replacements is enormously long. If you are appointed, what will you do to reduce it?'

'Nothing. I'm here for a colorectal job.'

Since the outcome of the appointments committee's deliberations should be preordained (see Plans A and B above), the only logical reason for its size is to spread the blame in the unlikely event a ne'er-do-well gets appointed.

In my case, I had three trials by sherry and three interviews from three applications. The first was for a DGH (district general hospital) north of London, a pleasant place close to open countryside with an old mate already working there who begged me to apply. Plan A prevailed and they appointed one of their former registrars, a talented and engaging woman who was well known on the circuit. She thoroughly deserved the job and we were all delighted for her. Sadly, not that many years later and while still in her prime, she developed cancer and died. The small world of vascular surgery was deeply saddened and dismayed at losing her.

The second interview was at a teaching hospital. I applied for the job because it was the thing to do, like a debutant coming out, attending every ball in town to display my assets and virtue. Every eligible vascular SR or Lecturer was shortlisted, perhaps five or six of us, and one already worked there. He happened to be another old mate from when we were both cutting our teeth in Sussex, so brazen curiosity was another motive. The tour of the hospital prior to the "trial by sherry" was disappointing. The facilities seemed lacklustre with a tiny ITU and much of the job leaning towards renal vascular work with transplants. Nick Scott, the incumbent, didn't need to join the tour but appeared for a sherry afterwards and said hello to me and the rest of us. He was in an invidious position, surrounded by competitors for a job he coveted and all but owned, except for the forthcoming interview in a few days' time. Yet we were all the same, had mirrored each other's career, trodden the same hard path, leapt the same hurdles, survived the brutally long hours, shared the elation of success and the deflation of failure. Over the years we'd met and drank beer, compared notes, tutored each other and learned in return. Vascular surgery had moulded us to an identical design, so any individual in that small circle of friends could do the job on offer without breaking a sweat. The one to clinch it would bring something else to the table, an intangible added value the others lacked. Yet whoever was appointed would get a heartfelt handshake and a sincere "Well done", free of any envy or malice.

Walking down the hill in the early evening sunshine to the nearest pub, I thought we looked like a group of Jehovah's Witnesses on our way to knock on doors and hand out The Watchtower, all smart suits, shiny shoes and haircuts. Nick wouldn't come for a drink after the trial by sherry finished. He said he had work to do, which was probably true – there's always something – but no doubt he also felt uncomfortable, knowing in all likelihood the job was in the bag (Plan A), while at the same time steeling himself for a huge upset caused by one of us.

Several beers later, we were all in agreement. If Nick wanted it, he was welcome to it. I'd already decided to look for a rural post, so it was no hardship. The job as described couldn't lure me back to the maelstrom of city life. Renal vascular with transplants implied sorting out transplant surgeons' cock-ups, and from what I'd seen of the specialty back then, it needed a lot of sorting. Most couldn't sew a button on a shirt, let alone one vessel to another, and it was full of starry-eyed adventurists with little talent, being flown or blue-lighted all over the country – especially exciting at night, guys – for organ harvesting. Not for me. I wanted a proper vascular post.

For differing reasons, the others voiced similar disenchantments. We were good, so why settle for second best?

'Should we turn up for the interview?' one asked.

'No choice,' we agreed. Having been shortlisted and given a glass of sherry, it would be rude and disrespectful to pull out. Besides, Nick deserved our support. Being the only candidate because the others have gone AWOL can't be good for morale. Let him get the job fairly and honestly, after an open, impartial, unbiased, competitive, and completely rigged interview.

A few days later I was at home in the kitchen, trying to conjure an extremely late lunch from the fridge. I'd been on call the previous night and consequently hadn't slept for thirty-six hours. My plan was to eat and crash out. The phone rang at about nine. From bitter experience, I knew it would be someone from the hospital asking for advice, or worse, my presence. A dozen possibilities came to mind, including that day's aneurysm. Perhaps it was bleeding? When I left the place only an hour before, everything was under control. Sod it, I simply had to answer, reasoning I'd get no rest either way. Grabbing the handset from its cradle on the wall, I groaned 'Hello,' into the mouthpiece, my voice laced with undertones of despair and sheer weariness.

'Well, I must say, that's a fine way to greet someone.'

I recognised the voice immediately, one of my previous chiefs from Sussex. I'd seen him intermittently at conferences over the years and we'd loosely kept in touch. A brilliant teacher and superb surgeon, I adored the man, as did all his registrars. 'Sorry about that. I thought it was work. Anyway, hello again, how are you?'

'I'm well, thank you, but it seems you've had a bad day.'

'Not bad, just long.'

We chatted amicably for a few minutes before he came to the point. 'Now, listen carefully. I rang because I've a little proposition for you.'

'Okay, fire away.' I was expecting an invitation to give a lecture to his local surgical club or some such. Filling an annual programme with relevant up-to-date speakers is difficult and I'd helped out previously. There was always a good meal in it.

'Before beginning, I want you to know I've just had exactly the same conversation with Nick Scott.'

'That's a coincidence – oddly enough, I saw him earlier this week, but carry on.' I was eager to know the plot. *Perhaps he's after a double act from two of his old boys? That'd be fun, the three of us having a slap-up meal and drink together.*

'You're being interviewed tomorrow for a job at my old alma mater. The word is it's between you and Nick. Whichever one of you doesn't get appointed, I'd like him to come here. There's a job ready and waiting for one of you, and we'd be absolutely delighted to have either. Nick agrees it's a fine plan and wants to do it. What do you think? If you lose out tomorrow, you come to us. If Nick loses, he comes.

After all, you could both do a lot worse.'

Momentarily stunned, it took me several seconds to respond. 'How on earth do you know any of this?'

'Oh, you know I can't divulge my sources. Nick asked me the same question and I gave him the same answer. Let's just call it consultant privilege, but this conversation is between you and me and mustn't go any further.'

'Fine, but answer this one. What happens if neither of us gets the job?'

'Short of a catastrophe, it's not going to happen. Nick asked me that as well. Honestly, you two are like peas in a bloody pod. I obviously taught both of you far too well,' he chuckled to himself. 'Now then, what do you say? If you can't decide right now that's okay, but at least consider it and let me know soon.'

'No need: my answer is yes. I think your plan is perfect and thank you very much for considering us.'

'Splendid. Now I can push on with things at this end. Good luck for tomorrow by the way. Whichever one of you they choose, we're all going to be winners.'

'Thanks for that, but I'm certain Nick will get the job, so it'll be me coming to you.'

'Yeah, yeah, yeah. Are you sure you're not both related?'

'Eh? What do you mean?'

'Nick said exactly the same thing about you.'

I still didn't sleep, but at least I was awake in my own bed. The conversation kept re-running in my mind. A firm offer of a job in my old stomping ground, and it felt ... delicious.

There was no other word to describe it. Including medical school, it had taken seventeen long years to get to the point where I could be my own boss. The time was right, and I was ready for it. Apart from tomorrow's interview for a job I didn't want, there was nothing else on the horizon. Jack Walters' post at King's would be advertised before long, but I wouldn't be applying. The hospital, the surgical unit and the staff were all fabulous, but the district was a dangerous hostile dump. I wanted me and my young family out of London. And my wish had just been granted.

But would a DGH post fulfil and satisfy me? I'd never harboured any ambition other than to become the best surgeon I could be. Fame and fortune, not commonly found within the world of medicine, never interested me. Yet academia gently tickled my intellect to the point where published research papers and articles were now the currency of my worth. More than that, they bestowed a kind of immortality in print. Would I miss it all? Possibly. But a teaching hospital isn't the sole repository of all scholarly thoughts; I'd find something to occupy my mind. There were positives to consider as well, like putting down permanent roots, not changing jobs and hospitals every five minutes, getting a decent house and staying put, no more on-call bedrooms, no more bleeps.

After a restless night, the morning rush-hour traffic was its usual constipated shitfest, yet for the first time I was glad of it. Knowing I would soon be escaping forever filled me with a serene clarity. I thumped the steering wheel in celebration. Yes! The Sussex job was the right one for me.

Plan A and B had worked their magic. All I needed now was to get through that day's interview without getting myself appointed.

The panel was as expected. Managers, a host of consultants (I knew the surgeons), a woman in a big hat, and wouldn't you know it, my old bête noir, Smiling Death himself, the external representative for the College. They all sat in a horseshoe arrangement facing me at one end – standard stuff, but intimidating if you weren't expecting it. The hat was directly opposite me, expensively flamboyant with a huge brim casting an even bigger shadow. Sadly, the lady camping out beneath it looked nothing like Audrey Hepburn.

There can't be many people who've faced an interview for a job they don't want, but believe me, it's a highly amusing experience. Particularly so, when you know the whole thing is a charade. But it was necessary to ensure they didn't favour me above my preferred candidate, Nick. Without a care in the world I thoroughly enjoyed myself, being careful to give answers that were just wide of the mark, sufficiently off the wall to rank me as eccentric but not entirely mad.

'When would you *not* operate on a leaking aneurysm?'

'In a teaching hospital I'd operate on them all, whatever the age or co-morbidity. The juniors need the practice.' *That answer still makes me wince.*

'What would you do to reduce the varicose vein waiting list?' *This from the hat.*

'Varicose veins should not be done on the NHS. Symptoms can be treated with elastic stockings prescribed by a GP. And the vast majority are women wanting corrective cosmetic surgery, so they should seek treatment in the private sector. To answer your question, I wouldn't add to the list by putting any more on it. As for those already waiting for an operation, your question is best directed to the surgeon they belong to.'

Smiling Death was quite charming. Over the years since my MS interrogation and beyond, I came to know the man better and grew to like him a lot. Despite the nickname, he was a nice guy who eventually became President of the College, and later still accepted a Knighthood. At the interview, he asked about research and my opinion on a recently published paper in which we shared an interest. But I sensed he'd cottoned on to our game when he gave me a surreptitious nod of approval.

As planned, and to everyone's delight, Nick got the job. He was always the right man for it. Soon afterwards I had my third interview, was duly appointed, and escaped from London for good. I couldn't have been happier.

We moved – me, my wife and baby girl – to a modest house on the edge of a pleasant small town. It had a large garden backing on to farmland with open countryside, and fulfilled my immediate idyll. From there both pursued our respective professional careers, were blessed with another baby girl, employed childminders, nannies and cleaners, sent the girls to a private school, moved to another house again, and again, until finally arriving in our forever home, a charming centuries-old manor house covered in wisteria, with acres of land, a horse, a couple of cats, a dog, an Aga in the farmhouse kitchen, and a huge yet affordable mortgage. The Liverpool docker's grandson had finally arrived. But it was tough. My wife was often away on business in the US or Europe, sometimes for over a week at a time, and though we synchronised diaries and I swapped my on-call duties, our two girls were infrequently parked in the theatre coffee room, still in their school uniforms and doing homework, while I attended to some early evening emergency. During those times, I discovered the easy option of feeding children at burger, fried chicken, or pizza houses, and learned – usually late on Sunday after they were both asleep in bed – that pleated school skirts are almost impossible to iron. Nor did I master the arcane art of plaiting long hair to either of my daughters' satisfaction. On schooldays, a ponytail held in an elastic band had to suffice.

Thirteen years after becoming a consultant, I was divorced, emotionally and financially broken, and living in a one-bedroom rented flat. The forever happy home proved to be a chaotic delusion, the breakup protracted, painfully sad, and deeply depressing. It took several years to fully recover, but when it was all over, when the self-loathing and guilt and despair had finally eaten their fill of my spirit, I found some sort of tranquil stability and made peace with myself. Throughout it all, my steadfast mistress, Surgery, stood by me. She was always my first love.

All parents, it seems, damage their children. We cannot help it. And that is my deepest regret. Perhaps this premise is the true core of the pseudo-philosophical religious claptrap of "Original sin". Consensual sex of itself cannot be sinful, but how the product is nurtured invariably is. No doubt many poets and writers have published their thoughts on this shameful cycle, but for me, two stand out.

Philip Larkin expressed it brutally in *This Be The Verse*: "They fuck you up, your mum and dad ..." And Mitch Albom, an American writer, likened a child to pristine glass, absorbing the prints of its handlers: "Some parents smudge, others crack, a few shatter childhoods completely into jagged little pieces, beyond repair."

My two baby girls are now full-grown women. Please forgive my fuck-ups, smudges, or worse. I've never stopped loving you.

In the autumn of 2011, at the age of fifty-nine, with twenty-four years as a consultant behind me and the prospect of retirement a distant speck on the horizon, I became aware of the lifetime pension pot allowance. A newspaper article announced it was to reduce, the following financial year, from £1.8 million to £1.5 million – sums of money way beyond my means or imagination. 'Well, that'll give the super-rich a headache,' I thought idly, before moving on to the crossword. But there in the first paragraph of the article, I spotted the word "surgeon" and it piqued my interest.

It explained that moderately high earners, like surgeons, would be particularly hard hit by the new rules. The "pot" wasn't a huge nest egg of millions stashed away in some pension fund to provide a retirement income from the interest it earned – as I imagined – but a multiple of the annual pension received. So, a work pension multiplied by a nominal life expectancy of 25 years could amount to a fair bit. Add the final lump sum to the pot, plus whatever a meagre personal pension might deliver, again similarly multiplied, and the total sum could be quite enormous, even though it would never exist as cash in the bank. Certain it couldn't possibly apply to yours truly, I nevertheless called my accountant for reassurance.

Yep, he said, after some quick back-of-a-fag-packet calculations, the article could have been written explicitly for me. He then went on to explain if I didn't retire before the next financial year, the taxman would eventually want around £150,000 from me.

'WHAT? You of all people know I don't have that sort of money.'

'Oh, don't worry, I'm sure he'll be happy to deduct it from your pension.'

'Bloody hell. What should I do?'

'It's your life and your decision, but if it were me, I'd get out now. The lifetime allowance is bound to shrink further, so if you stay working, our friends at HMRC will eventually demand even more of your hard-earned spondulicks when you finally do retire. It's really a no-brainer.' Similar discussions involving surgeons, both older and younger than me, were happening all over the country.

The following spring, I retired early, as did many of my contemporaries, driven out by the taxman. At a stroke, the law of unintended consequences robbed the NHS of its most senior surgical workhorses. Some, after a statutory period of absence, returned part-time on short-term contracts, mainly in teaching or managerial posts. Most didn't. All that talent, wisdom and experience was lost forever.

I didn't go cold turkey. Private practice and some sessions at a nearby community hospital to help with their waiting list kept me moderately busy and fed my addiction to patients and surgery for a couple of years, but by then the lure of complete freedom and the promise of summer weaned me off the habit. One Thursday evening in April 2014, I snapped the briefcase shut and brought my final clinic to an end. After a lifetime in medicine, it was time to walk away. There were no regrets.

Well, almost none. Once accustomed to the gentle pace of a comfortable retirement, I began to miss the patients, the camaraderie of colleagues, the mental stimulation, the challenges, the gossip, the sheer fun of it all. But what I didn't miss was the constant stone-in-shoe angst of being on call day and night for an emergency, or the worry and concern over a sick patient, particularly when it was a child. After many decades of uncomfortable companionship, the stone was suddenly gone, notable only by its absence. I'd lost an irritating old friend whose existence was never fully appreciated. One who ensured I was always up early for work but accompanied me through countless sleepless nights, who kept me sharp and alert even when my exhausted body craved rest, and made me forever vigilant, careful to check and re-check, again, and again. The period of mourning lasted many months, but in time, my step became lighter and carefree as I learned to live without its nagging presence. It felt like a new beginning, a new life. And I could never go back.

So, what to do now? A good start would be to eliminate the possibility of doctoring again. I phoned the General Medical Council to tell them I'd retired, wouldn't be paying my annual registration fee – around £400 or more – and they could now remove me from the register.

'You can't retire like that,' said the twelve-year-old at the other end.

'What do you mean, I can't? I already have.'

'We can't de-register you without proof you've stopped working and that your employer has no outstanding issues going back five years.'

'Outstanding issues? Such as?'

'Broadly speaking: fitness to practise and ongoing litigation.'

'I don't have any outstanding issues.'

'We have no proof of that.'

'And if I don't pay my fee, what will you do?'

'You'll be struck off.'

'But that's what I want.'

The rest of the exchange was equally bizarre. As I

understood it, the GMC doesn't want doctors withdrawing from practice and fleeing the country in order to avoid impending medico-legal proceedings. They would much rather absconders clear it with them first. Huh? Accordingly, I couldn't retire, or abscond, unless my sheet was clean. For almost forty years the only interest they'd ever shown in me was financial, but now alert to my situation, they were going to cling like a tick until I complied with their demands. In the end, troubled by visions of epaulettes, gold buttons and medal ribbons being cut off with a sword, I conceded defeat and agreed to an honourable discharge rather than the other sort.

'I'll send you a form for your hospital to complete.'

'I'll need four.'

Soon afterwards, I received an anonymous thank-you card, forwarded to me from the main hospital. It served as a poignant reminder of the enormously rewarding job I've had the privilege and good luck to spend my life doing, and of the people who really mattered, the patients. It was a small card, about three by three inches, but its handwritten message packed a punch.

'Hello, you won't remember me, but over twenty years ago when I was a young woman, you did an operation to cure my sweaty hands. It changed my life completely and gave me the confidence to succeed. I'm now director of a Fortune 500 company. So, thank you and enjoy your retirement.'

I did the rather technical operation on dozens of similar patients back then, before injections of Botox took over.

Nearly all of them were young women, so even if I could track down the notes of every single one, it would be a futile search and leave me no wiser as to the identity of my well-wisher, which is as it should be. Nevertheless, she must be well connected to have learned of my retirement, as well as being thoughtful, caring and kind. Whoever you are, thanks for the card and the message. It meant a great deal to me.

Now it's my turn. Thank you to all the many thousands of patients who changed my life for the better. Your courage showed me the indomitable resilience of the human spirit. Your trust instilled humility and a determination to do my best. Your recovery gave me joy. And even in those dark miserable times when things weren't going well, when I thought I'd failed you and felt like slinking away to hide my shame in some dark secluded cave, you gave me the will and strength to stand by your bedside each day, checking the charts, assessing your progress, tweaking the medication. Though you never knew it, I always added a good dose of my own sheer willpower with a surreptitious touch of your hand or forearm, coupled with a silent wish. 'By tomorrow, you'll be better.'

EPILOGUE

I smoke too much, drink too much, eat too much, don't do enough exercise, shave when the stubble itchiness forces me to, dress like a shambling vagrant, can't believe the crap that passes for daytime TV entertainment, use BBC Radio 4 as background white noise, buy *The Telegraph* for the Matt cartoon, letters page and crossword, live in a small isolated rural home, do a bit of gardening when the sun shines, botch occasional DIY jobs, and think all teenagers should have their smartphones impounded in their rectum at mealtimes. And whereas it was work that once motivated me to get out of bed ridiculously early each morning, now it's my bladder. My wife – I remarried a few years ago – calls me a lazy git, despite reassurances I'm simply pacing myself to prolong our time together and make her happy. The dog, a black lab, doesn't venture an opinion on my behaviour, though in the lazy git stakes he beats me paws down, snoozing all day on the sofa or bed, except for greeting the postman and demanding food or walks: we must be soulmates. Yes, I'm a fully paid up member of the happily retired curmudgeon club and for six years have been content as a pig in shit. The one thing that disturbs this blissful porcine existence, has me brushing off one of my well-saved suits, polishing my shoes and getting a haircut, is the need to attend funerals. Most are for work colleagues I've known for decades – surgeons, anaesthetists and the very occasional half-decent physician, all as close to me as any family – and they're popping off with alarming frequency.

Medical funerals have a different dynamic to others I attend. Having spent a career dealing hands-on or wrist-deep with every intimate aspect of thousands of lives and hundreds of deaths, I suppose we become insensitive to the usual emotions associated with these traditionally mournful gatherings. Rather than shedding useless tears over the inevitable, we whisper post-mortem questions: 'What did he die from? Who looked after him? Mode of death? Was she in pain? Lose her dignity?' And especially, 'Who fucked up?' In large part, that's the reason we go, to ensure no negligence or fuck-ups. Either would be a shameful betrayal of one of our own, by one of our own, and taint us all with guilt for not getting more involved. Once assured our friend died well, it's drinks all round, a communal catch-up with handshakes and hugs, and see you next time.

This one's at a bleakly efficient crematorium, befitting an unpretentious man who scorned religion and faced terminal malignancy with the same calm logic he navigated through life. In the front row, nearest the wreath-adorned coffin with obligatory photo, his wife is flanked by their three children, the oldest with a handwritten eulogy stowed like a leaden weight within her clutch bag. I knew them as kids, playing in the garden with my own at countless summer barbeques and birthday parties, and operated on one of them. Now, they're all grown into adulthood at the same relative speed, while the rest of us, contrary to the laws of physics, have somehow accelerated into senility and are dropping like flies. The body in the coffin belonged to a matchless gasman and even better friend, always willing to lend a hand or give sound advice, and expect the same of me, day or night. I shall miss him, and he would call me a bloody fool for doing so. Scattered around the middle rows with me are other old friends, each nursing similar memories and wondering how long it'll be before one of us becomes the star attraction. At the rear are fresher faces, come from afar to pay respects to their one-time boss. Later, at the reception with a beer or white wine in hand, they'll swap tales of the anaesthetic maxims he drilled into them and smile as each confesses a strict observance to his truths.

When the secular celebrant – a large, improbably cheerful lady with curiously butter-blonde hair, heavy make-up, and a green trouser suit in which her backside would be Exhibit A in a fashion-crime court case – calls us to order, I stop scanning, adopt a suitably reverential pose and immediately start daydreaming. It must be close to a dozen by now, and if I survive long enough, a dozen more to go. Some have been short and simple like today, others grandiose with high-ranking clergy, a rousing organ, pealing bells, incense, altar boys, and a choir belting out everyone's favourite hymns. Most are somewhere in between. Is the degree of funerary indulgence a measure of self-importance, belief in the unknowable, or a reflection of the esteem, shame, love or loathing felt by those who pay for it? No matter, it's an idle muse of little worth.

Now, my thoughts turn to the young people at the back, the next generation of torchbearers for anaesthesia. They're a constant feature at all medical funerals: different people, different specialties, but acolytes all the same, and half a lifetime ago I was one of them, paying homage to my own surgical chiefs after their flame had extinguished. With a sudden insight, I realise this same scenario has played out for millennia.

At the heart of this gathering, lies an ancient medical fellowship of teaching and learning to which I was previously blind. Only another doctor knows the torment, the terror, the soul-searching, the desolate heartbreak and the glorious joy doctoring can bring. Only another doctor knows the ultimate futility of the craft. And only another doctor can show you how to bear it.

Though we are here to salute a friend, a colleague and a mentor, we also honour the memory of every medic who ever lived. Just as it should be. As it ever was. Through time and history, the same continuous thread connects us all.

ACKNOWLEDGEMENTS

My many patients unknowingly conceived this book, but other people assisted its gestation. Most paid the cost by reading one of the numerous drafts and suggesting changes. You have only yourselves to blame. Love and heartfelt thanks to:

The wise Lady Di, for hooking me from the depths, putting up through thick and thin with what she landed, and eventually agreeing to marry me.

Brilliant Clare, my darling baby sister. Many years separate us, but we're cut from the same granite.

Howard, Ian and Tony of the annual Annan fishing trip, who've kept me grounded, side-splittingly entertained and very inebriated for more years than I care to remember.

Ian and Chris, and Bernie and Liz, stalwart friends and loyal colleagues for most of my life, who insisted I delete much of the foul language.

Harry and Len, who taught me life and surgery. I'll forever be in your debt.

Polly and Pete, our lovely learned neighbours.

Colin, a talented fellow aviator and insightful critic.

And Bailey, the faithful and gentlemanly hound, who

listened to every iteration during our long walks, and sadly is looking as old as I feel.

Finally, my scribbles would never have seen the light of day without the help, encouragement, and editorial precision of Stephanie Hale and her excellent team at Powerhouse Publications. Thank you for being my champion and guru. I'm willing to bet the contents of your cutlery, knicker and sock drawers look like soldiers on parade. Furthermore, I promise never to pen the word "which" ever again.

THE AUTHOR

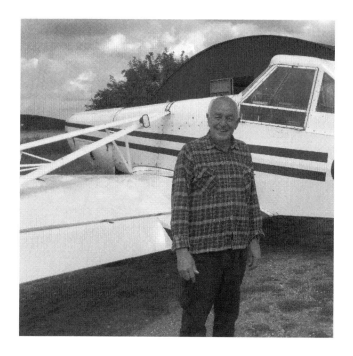

The author attended The Middlesex Hospital Medical School, London, and qualified as a doctor in 1975. After post-graduate training in a succession of hospitals in and around the capital he was appointed as a consultant general and vascular surgeon in 1987.

In 2014, he retired to rural Cambridgeshire with his wife, a dog, two ducks, and a horse. When he's not repairing broken posts and rails, or mowing paddocks, he flies gliders and is also a tug pilot, pulling gliders into the sky behind an ancient Pawnee.

During his medical career, he was a passionate teacher and trainer, co-authoring two textbooks and numerous scientific papers. This is his first book for the interested general reader.

Printed in Great Britain
by Amazon